Not Another

Guide to Stress in General Practice!

Second edition

Edited by
David Haslam

Radcliffe Medical Press

Radcliffe Medical Press Ltd
18 Marcham Road, Abingdon, Oxon OX14 1AA

First edition 1994

British Library Cataloguing in Publication Data

A catalogue record for this book is available from the British Library.

ISBN 1 85775 446 8

Typeset by Joshua Associates Ltd, Oxford
Printed and bound by TJ International Ltd, Padstow, Cornwall

Contents

Preface

What is going on? Why are GPs becoming so obsessed with their own stress? Do GPs really have a worse time than the rest of the population? And why is every medical newspaper full of reports on stress, advice on how to survive and tragic tales of suicide in the medical profession? What has happened to general practice? Indeed, is there really a problem at all? Has stress simply become fashionable? Have GPs moved from being stiff upper lipped pillars of their local communities to pathetic whingers?

The idea for this book was originally conceived at a retreat for members of the East Anglia Faculty of the Royal College of General Practitioners (RCGP). It was felt that doctors needed positive guidance on how to get through the stresses that seem to affect almost every GP. At the meeting anecdotes abounded. We all felt under pressure. We all knew colleagues who were under tremendous strain, marriages and partnerships that were not surviving and the depth of misery felt by so many doctors. From my own experience as a writer in the medical press, I had found that every time I wrote a piece about stress, I would get letters from doctors that I had never met expressing their sheer despair and their relief that someone was writing publicly about the way that they felt.

When I began to contact colleagues for their help in writing this book, I did not expect to discover the sheer scale of stress in our branch of the profession. Nearly three-quarters of the doctors that I spoke to had received treatment for depression – whether with counselling, formal psychotherapy or medication. Everyone else either had a practice that had been affected by a partner suffering from severe stress, or had other close connections with stressed GPs. Not a single doctor denied that stress was a major problem – it had permeated almost every practice. General practice is facing dreadful workforce problems, and stress is one of the main reasons for the poor recruitment and early retirement that greatly exacerbates these difficulties.

Every GP needs to understand stress. This book explores some of the causes of stress, looks at case histories, specific problems, stressed practices, the particular stresses that face women doctors and will give help and advice to aid in the recovery of every GP from the battering that we all feel we have been under. Every author of every chapter is a GP. No one understands this job quite like we do. I hope and believe that it will be helpful.

David Haslam
May 2000

Note: Whilst PCGs are referred to throughout the book, it is realised that other primary care organisations apply in Scotland, Wales and Northern Ireland – however, the principles involved are exactly the same.

List of contributors

Tina Ambury
GP Locum
Bushey and Watford

Liz Bingham
General Practitioner
Newbury, Berks

Simon Brown
General Practitioner
Ramsey, Cambridgeshire

IK Campbell
General Practitioner
Snettisham, Norfolk

Tom Davies
General Practitioner
Yaxley, Cambridgeshire

Andrew Eastaugh
General Practitioner
Southwold, Suffolk

David Haslam
General Practitioner
Ramsey, Cambridgeshire

Kevork Hopayian
General Practitioner
Leiston, Suffolk

John Mitchell
General Practitioner
Stamford, Lincolnshire

Paul Sackin
General Practitioner
Alconbury, Cambridgeshire

Sidha Sambandan
General Practitioner
Norwich, Norfolk

George Smerdon
General Practitioner
St Ives, Cambridgeshire

Kate Wishart
General Practitioner
King's Cliffe, Northants

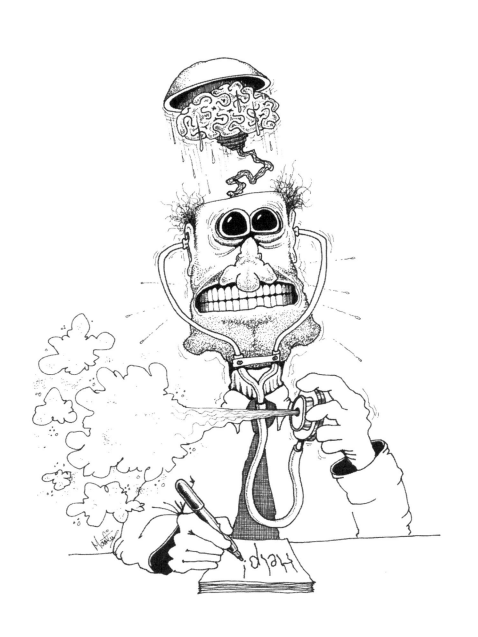

1 Introduction: a personal view on stress in general practice

David Haslam

Every medical student is taught about stress. We learn about the physiological and biochemical definitions of stress and develop some understanding of what happens at the cellular level. Understanding stress in behavioural terms is very much harder. It is rather like the hippopotamus – easy to recognise but extraordinarily difficult to describe.

The excellent RCGP Occasional Paper on *Stress Management in General Practice* offers three different definitions of stress.[1] The first of these is the Oxford English Dictionary's stimulus-based definition: to subject (a material thing, a bodily organ, a mental faculty) to stress or strain; to overwork, fatigue. We all would certainly recognise this definition. In recent years, GPs have been given more and more to do. No one ever tells us what we can stop doing to release more time for the new activity. More and more is added into the workload, until finally 'the piece of straw breaks the camel's back'.

The second definition is response-based and considers the physiological response to stress. Here the alarm reaction triggers autonomic responses as the body attempts to deal with the stress. Obviously, if there is too much stress, the body simply cannot take any more and becomes exhausted. All too many GPs have battled on, attempting to cope with stress, until exhaustion or collapse occurs. What happens at the cellular level, also happens at the human level.

The final definition looks at stress as a dynamic process, taking into account the external stress and the characteristics of the person becoming stressed. One such definition states that stress is 'a particular relationship between the person and the environment that is appraised by the person as taxing or exceeding his or her resources and endangering his or her wellbeing'.[2] This dynamic view implies that stress can occur if there is an imbalance between an individual's perceived strengths and resources, and the demands on his or her time and skills. What may be stressful for one GP may be enjoyable and refreshing for another. It is the individual who counts.

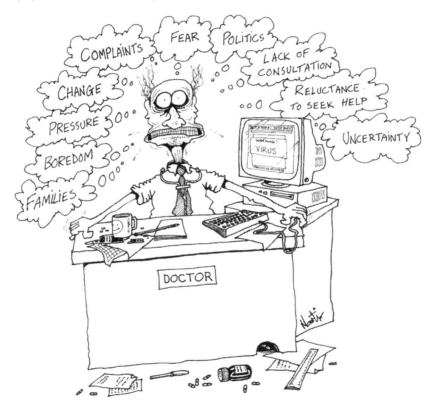

What makes GPs stressed?

Why should GPs be so prone to stress? Compared to the vast majority of the population, GPs are relatively well paid, well respected and secure; few of us face redundancy. Almost every study of the public's perceptions of professional groups puts GPs at the top, even in these post-Bristol inquiry days. We are generally trusted and mostly admired.

So what is it about our jobs that makes us so tense and can drive an extraordinary number of us to drink, drugs, marital breakdown and suicide? In the spring of 1993, the Secretary of State for Health, Virginia Bottomley, gave the introductory address at a conference on the 'Prevention of Suicide'. In this, she advocated a policy to reduce stress in the workforce in order to reduce the number of lives lost through suicide.

Fine words. Great intentions. However, four of the occupational groups most likely to commit suicide are doctors, dentist, veterinary surgeons and pharmacists; the Department of Health should perhaps have more than an academic interest in this topic. Indeed, perhaps it should recognise that less-stressed GPs are going to offer a better service to their patients.

Time management

A few years ago I was feeling very stressed. I initially assumed that it was because of the pressure and responsibilities of the job. A non-medical friend had pointed out how he would find it impossible to live with the life-and-death decisions that GPs make as second nature. I had assumed that it was these stresses that were causing me problems.

However, after reading a basic book on stress management, I took its advice and kept a stress diary for a week. This was simplicity itself. Every hour, on the hour, I wrote down how stressed I felt on a scale of 0 (totally relaxed) to 10 (desperately tense). If the score had changed by a factor of two or more, either up or down, I wrote down why.

Was it the life-and-death decisions that stressed me? Not a chance. It was time pressure, which was most often unnecessary.

For example, I had set myself a target of doing my visits before lunch, and having lunch at one o'clock. If I was late for lunch I felt stressed. If I was late doing a visit, patients would say, 'I thought you were never coming!' and this implied criticism then stressed me even more.

The solution to this was simple. If I was busy, my receptionist would phone the patient and say, 'Dr Haslam is rather busy. He'll be in this afternoon'. Simple. Successful. And you might think rather absurdly obvious!

Can things like time pressure really be a major cause of stress? In fact, numerous studies have shown that time management is the biggest single factor that GPs can change to reduce their stress at work. Overrunning surgeries, insufficient appointment times, interruptions during consultations and failure to deal with paperwork efficiently are all aspects of our lives that we can tackle. In particular, research has shown clearly that patient-centred doctors who issue fewer prescriptions and do more listening tend to become stressed. Part of the reason for this may lie in the fact that listening takes time, taking time leads to overrunning surgeries, and patients who have to wait for a long time tend to increase the GP's levels of stress even further.

Of course, what is stressful for me may not be stressful for you. But be aware that you might be wrong about what you think is stressful for you. It really is worth undertaking a simple study, such as keeping a stress diary, to find out what makes you stressed.

Other potential causes of stress

In addition to time management, there are a number of specific problems that could be important factors in the stresses you suffer in your working life. These could include the following:

Complaints

There can be little doubt that the increase in complaints against GPs is causing enormous stress for many doctors. Patients are being encouraged to complain more and more. Liz Bingham worked as GP advisor to the NHS Ombudsman, and her chapter in this book helps bring a fresh view on this distressing topic.

Change

Everything keeps changing. Not only from an organisational point of view, but also from a clinical point of view. It seems that almost every week, some aspect of our job is shown to be useless or in need of change. Highly motivated, slightly obsessional GPs may begin to despair when informed that an aspect of care they have laboured hard over is useless and does not improve patient outcome.

Pressure

Every week the medical press contains articles encouraging GPs to do more or to do better. We are criticised for our handling of almost everything, from backache to infertility and from depression to Alzheimer's disease. Articles appear showing how we can set up a clinic for this, that and usually the other as well – without telling us what we can stop doing in order to liberate the time for these 'improved' services. We need to learn how to say 'no'.

Political

Rationing, primary care groups (PCGs), and never-ending organisational change, tied with the way that we have become agents for a state system, rather than independent doctors who simply try to do the best for our patients, has deeply distressed many GPs. The government has tried insidiously to expand the GP's traditional role. We are putting ourselves more and more in the position of being made to accept the blame for the failures of the NHS. PCGs are a brilliant concept, for the government, which lead to the centralisation of credit, but the devolution of blame.

Lack of consultation

The imposition of changes to the way we work by the government has not been a success. All experts on management point out that consultation on change is essential. I believe that in years to come the imposition of many recent NHS changes will be taught world-wide as an example of how not to run a business. And those of us at the sharp end still have to face the sick, worried and unhappy people every day – and I don't just mean our colleagues.

Fear

More and more doctors feel stressed by the threat of violence from their patients, either in the surgery or on visits – especially at night. They are frightened of assault, but face an internal conflict if they are reluctant to visit after a callout request.

Boredom

Many doctors become bored or frustrated by the apparent same-ness of so much general practice. One surgery can seem very much like every other, and the future can offer no excitement. The lack of a career structure to general practice does not help, so we have to create our own. This may involve developing a special clinical interest, writing, researching or teaching. One colleague wrote an MD thesis on back pain and turned a routine task into academic achievement. There are opportunities, but we do have to create them ourselves.

Uncertainty

In their wisdom, our medical schools chose us because we got good science 'A' levels. We are now in jobs where scientific certainty is rare. How many diagnoses are you totally certain about? How many management plans are free from debate and full of scientific fact? Indeed, are the very people who become GPs those who are least equipped to live with the pressure of the job? It is essential that we should be able to tolerate uncertainty. Many of us can't.

Families

There can be real pressure in attempting to combine general practice with family life. Is the good doctor one who drops everything to help a patient in distress, for whom nothing is too much trouble and who visits terminally ill patients even on days off? Or is this a recipe for disaster, for burnout, for resentful children or for divorce? Getting the balance right can be enormously stressful. When I was a houseman, my registrar gave me a good piece of advice: 'Never accept any definition of off-duty that doesn't allow you to become blind drunk. It's not that you will ever want to get drunk, but if you can't then you aren't off duty'.

Reluctance to seek help

GPs tend to be more isolated than hospital doctors, and can be professionally lonely. However, when we have problems, we rarely own up to them. Professor Sydney Brandon, as Chairman of the National Counselling Service for Sick Doctors, commented that GPs 'often have very great guilt at assuming the patient role and are reluctant to seek treatment. The GP often registers himself with a close colleague and is reluctant to face that colleague when he is under par'.[3]

A study comparing the health and lifestyles of GPs and teachers, both of whom have had to face imposed changes that have caused widespread dissatisfaction, stated 'the frequency of reported mental health problems in both professions gives cause for concern'.[4] We owe it to ourselves, our partners and our families to take care of ourselves. Also we all have GPs registered with us. Do we really offer them the care that they deserve?

Conclusion

Despite this catalogue of problems, I believe that general practice can be one of the most stimulating jobs in the world. When it goes well, there is simply nothing to beat it. When it goes badly, it beats us. This book will show some of the ways that you can survive – from keeping physically fit to understanding your stress, and from caring for yourself to caring for colleagues. I hope you find it of real value.

References

1   Royal College of General Practitioners (1993) *Stress Management in General Practice.* Occasional Paper 61. Royal College of General Practitioners, London.

2   Lazarus RS and Folkman S (1984) *Stress, Appraisal and Coping.* Springer Verlag, New York.

3   Agnew T (1993) Doctors crack under pressure. *Gen Prac.* **April 9**: 49.

4   Chambers R and Belcher J (1993) Comparison of the health and lifestyle of general practitioners and teachers. *Br J Gen Pract.* **43**: 378–82.

2 Recognising and responding to stress

Andrew Eastaugh

You see doctor, life is so stressful having to cope with the dogs without any help. I've told George that I can't run the London house as well. What I need is a jolly good rest, so I've booked into The Swan for a week but if you could give me my usual prescription, I'd know I was all right.

She was about 55, well dressed, well padded, well connected and very well heeled. It was Friday afternoon. I had been on a '1 in 2' in a flu epidemic that had hit everyone, including my family. The one thing focused in my sights was a very large gin to start a weekend off-duty. Sounds familiar?

So what is this stress thing that everyone is going on about? Who was stressed, me or the patient? And how are we trying to cope? Mrs Double-Barrelled is in fact a bi-polar depressive with very thick notes, who has learnt, often painfully, what she can and cannot cope with. She has imposed limits on her responsibilities and can recognise the signs of impending doom in time to take evasive action. In the modern jargon, she has learnt good stress management. The only pharmacological help she uses is given under medical direction.

On the other hand, I feel trapped into taking on more than I can cope with, to such an extent that I feel besieged and threatened by the people I am meant to be helping. The fact that Mrs Double-Barrelled can afford not to work and to stay in luxury hotels is certainly as convenient from her point of view, as the GP's contract and mode of working is idiotic from mine, and this only serves to illustrate that stress management must be built out of practical reality, rather than idealistic fantasy.

Following on from WC Fields's saying, 'A man who hates dogs and children can't be wholly bad', some stress is beneficial. If life was totally without stress it would be boring and pointless. In fact a lack of stressors may induce stress by the sheer effect of under-stimulation. Human performance behaves according to Starling's Law of the Heart: as the strain increases, output correspondingly increases to an optimum range. After that the coping mechanisms become overstretched and performance falls (Figure 2.1). Just as the dilated heart has to beat harder and faster to deal with the ever-increasing load, the overstretched doctor has to work harder and faster to stay in the same place before finally burning out, often drowning in an alcoholic fluid overload. So if you feel in need of a large dose of stress-relieving furosemide, read on.

Recognising stress

So what is stress? How do I know I've got it and what can I do about it? In engineering terms, stress is the result of a load

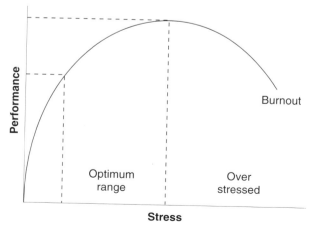

Figure 2.1   Effect of increasing stress on performance levels.

operating on a body. The effect it has is measurable in terms of strain, which results from the interaction of the stressor with the resilience of the body. In human stress, the picture is less clear-cut, partly because we cannot measure stress and partly because a force may be either a stressor or stress preventer, depending on how it is applied, how it relates to other forces and how the individual perceives it. This last factor is the real grounds of hope, for it is here that we can often influence things constructively.

A good way of thinking about it is as a pair of scales, with coping resources in one pan and stressors in the other (Figure 2.2). The balance of the scales depends not only on the relative weights in each pan but also the position of the pivot along the arm. This pivot point relates to the individual's own innate resources, how he or she views life and, in particular, what Kobasa *et al.* call 'hardiness'.[1] Recognising stress is like reading the scales.

- What are the stressors in the right-hand pan?
- What are my coping resources in the left-hand pan?
- Can I move the pivot point to the right to gain the maximum mechanical advantage?

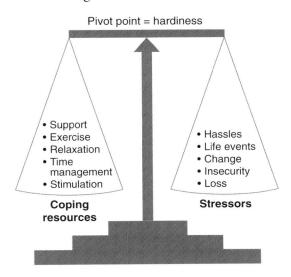

Figure 2.2   Balance between stressors and coping resources.

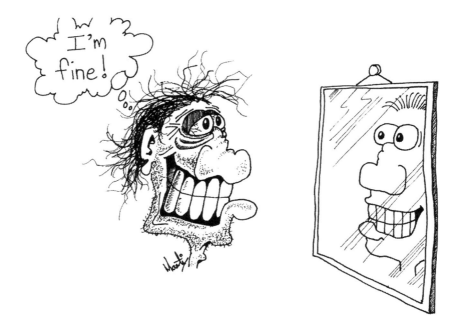

Stressors

Almost all major changes to our lives are stressors or potential stressors – probably because people are, by and large, conservative and easily frightened by the challenge and uncertainty of new situations. I found the 1990 GP Contract very stressful, not only because of the way it was introduced and the lack of proper trials and appraisal, but also because it challenged and changed something very central to my professional life: my role as a doctor. The usual benchmarks were being swept away and I was left feeling vulnerable.

These changes came not long after my father's death, which had affected me more than I had expected as he was 90 years old and had been ill for some time. These two major life events occurring together left me feeling quite undermined. It is not only the threats and perceived negative changes that act as stressors but also positive ones such as marriage. However, these positive events often bring with them their own built-in contribution to counterbalance the coping resources, by providing personal support and pleasure.

Most of the time it is not the sudden major life events that get to us, but the constant dripping of minor hassles plus the insidious creeping addition of extra work. There is almost a sense in which our ability to cope with the major stressors, such as a busy surgery, are proportional to our irritation at the minor ones, such as finding the coffee is cold when you get to it.

> . . . it's not the large things that send a man to the
> madhouse . . . death he's ready for, or murder, incest, robbery,
> fire, flood . . .
> no, it's the continuing series of small tragedies
> that send a man to the
> madhouse . . .
> not the death of his love
> but a shoelace that snaps
> with no time left . . .
>
> (From *The Shoelace*, © Charles Bukowski 1992,
> *Mockingbird Wish Me Luck*, Black Sparrow Press.)

For those who like lists and scores, there are numerous stressor rating scales to choose from.[2] Probably of greater practical value is to make a personal note of your current hassles and so realise the effect that these rather trivial occurrences are having on you. A stress diary is a good way of doing this (Table 2.1).[3] Identifying the situations and the feelings they engender allows for proper recognition of how you feel. The action taken may or may not be appropriate, but recording encourages reflection for future learning.

Coping resources

The antidote to hassles is prosaically known as 'uplifts', but I much prefer 'What makes your heart sing?'. Those things that give you a

Time	Situation	Feelings	Action
Table 2.1 An example of a stress diary			
8.45 a.m.	Anxious patient on telephone for ages	Bad start to the day, starting late	OK I'm late, so what
9.30	Heartsink patient No. 2	Oh no, not again!	Yet another referral
10.00	Appreciative patient	Feels good	OK, I'm not so bad after all
10.30	Recently bereaved young widow	Really sad	Need a break, get a coffee

lift, that give value and pleasure to your existence. The first few sunny days of March can lift the spirits and the prospect of the summer's sailing enlivens, what is for me, the drudgery of varnishing a boat. Just as it is possible to score the hassles of your day, so it can be worthwhile to note the things that have 'heart-sing' quality. Often the act of looking at life in this way can act as a cultivator and it is surprising how much of an otherwise bland day can be inspired to new heights. If in doubt, try looking for things that make your heart sing in your next surgery – it will probably help your patients as well.

It is crucial to realise that the operative word here is 'heart' not 'brain'. I cope better when I feel the sun on my skin and derive pleasure through it, and not just because I know it is there. One of the myriad of problems with the middle-class work ethic that has influenced many of us, especially in medicine, is the idea that feelings – and especially our own – are of little importance, and that pleasure is something to be had only on high days and holidays. That is not to advocate a life of selfish self-indulgence, but rather to give proper weight and priority to those things in life that hold true meaning.

This is not always as obvious as it seems, as it is not uncomon to find that things that we used to hold important or thought we did, no longer hold such relevance. The Life Line exercise is a useful way of standing back from the everyday hurly-burly to see if you are going where you want:

Birth _____ * _____ Death

Mark off where you think you are with an asterisk, and then look at what you have done with your life. Now think what you would like to have achieved by the time you get to the end? Are you heading in the right direction? Many of our frustrations arise from spending all our time on the 'oughts' of life, not on what we really want to achieve. Remember, life is not a dress rehearsal but is for real.

Support

Just as a lack of self-esteem and value creates a stressor climate, so does the sense of personal value and worth create a climate to cope with stress. For an individual the need to be loved, accepted and valued intrinsically is a basic requirement for self-actualisation.[4] Maslow, in his pyramidal hierarchy of needs puts it at the third level,[5] above the need for physiological satisfaction (hunger, thirst, etc.) and the need for safety. We can only develop this sense of belonging and love through others and what they can give us. Thus the support that we develop and receive is crucial to our fulfilment and our ability to cope with stress.

None of our relationships are ideal, and when they fail or are stretched, they move to the other side of the scales and become stressors. Thus we are left doubly disadvantaged. If all our support comes from one or two sources, such as our spouse and a colleague at work, the effects can be catastrophic should one or other fail us. Is there enough diversity in our support, or are we overdependent on one or two individuals? Lastly, do we think they are happy giving us this support and have we acknowledged the help they give us?

Education

As doctors and primary healthcare workers, we are in the business of giving support and listening to others, not only to our patients at the rate of one every 8–10 minutes, but also to our staff and other members of the team we lead. We can only give to others what we have received ourselves, but many doctors never get the opportunity to be on the receiving end of good active listening. We need to create opportunities to explore the problems we are encountering, to understand the personal and professional complexities of those problems, so that we can seek to address them. Systems of peer-supported learning, such as mentoring and co-tutoring, can enable us to turn the causes of our stress into educational opportunities that can often be remedied.[6] As shown earlier, stress frequently arises from our inability to cope with problems that we are encountering. If we can identify these problems, we can look for solutions or ways round them. Because stress is the result of our own personal dynamic interacting with situations, we need to develop understanding of ourselves, our reactions and our feelings in order to understand what is lying at the root of the problem. Peer support, particularly through active listening, empowers an individual's ability to reflect on his or her experience. The stress diary (Table 2.1) can go on to become the basis for an educational or professional development plan, by working on the problems to identify learning needs, educational action and, hopefully, new understanding or skills.[7]

Planning time effectively

How do you eat an elephant sandwich? . . . little by little. One of the most daunting feelings is that of being overwhelmed by tasks or responsibilities. Like the elephant sandwich, if we break tasks up into bite-sized pieces, they become manageable. Time management is the art of planning your available time according to the tasks you have to achieve, so as to make the best use of resources.

Somebody once said that the only thing predictable about general practice is its unpredictability. On the basis of this true, but misunderstood, statement, generations of GPs have been flying around their practices, late for everything, increasing either their patients', staff's, or their own stress, often all three. It is precisely because of the unpredictable nature of some of our work that we have to plan our time effectively and plan in space for the unpredictable, because we know it will happen. The trouble is not that we cannot cope with the urgent and emergency work, but because it is not allotted its space, it crowds out other work, as important but less instantaneously demanding. How many times in the last week or month have you been called away from something 'important and not urgent' to deal with 'something not important but urgent', only to find you have missed your original opportunity?

A common source of stress for GPs is the pressure of trying to keep on time in a surgery. Howie *et al.* found that GPs whose mean consultation time was longer than the mean booked time not only experienced more stress, but also consulted less effectively.[8] A time management approach to this is to determine your mean consultation time and make it the same as your booked consultation time. Inevitably, the unpredictable will occur and catch-up periods can also be allotted. While this will not eradicate the problem, it can reduce the magnitude of it, as well as provide the doctor with the knowledge and means to control the pressure.

Relaxation

We are all aware of the fright, fight or flight response – sympathetic nervous system racing to go, pupils dilated, heart rate up, skin circulation cut down, glucose stores mobilised, so that our ancestors could race away from the sabre-toothed tigers or other activities that required urgent physical exertion! Analogous to the excitation response is a relaxation response, which seems to have been forgotten until recently. Unfortunately, evolution, not having heard of targets or performance-related pay, has not managed to update our physiology to deal with the potential threats to '*Homo medicus*' posed by the introduction of primary care groups.

Nowadays, although most threats are mental or emotional rather than physical, they still produce the same physiological response, but only the mental alertness of the fright, fight or flight response is required. This often results in two things. First, we have an unsettled and racing mind that churns things over and over and, second our bodies lack the physical stimulus and exercise they need to burn off the adrenergic response. As part of monitoring your stress, take a look at your exercise and what you do to relax. By this I mean physiologically relaxing – not just a couple of beers in front of the television.

Moving the pivot point

The third factor governing the stress balance is the pivot point, which determines the mechanical advantage of one pan over the other on the scales. This is in many senses the key to the problem. Unlike mechanical stress, in the human variety cause and effect are not always clearly distinguishable. If things start to get stressful, I am less able to cope and they consequently get worse; conversely, the opposite applies. So many of the coping skills not only counterbalance the stressors, but also improve one's innate ability to handle stress.

People who are resilient to stress tend to exhibit the three Cs, which together form what has been called 'hardiness'.[1]

- **Commitment** is a tendency to involve oneself in life and one's activities. Committed people have a sense of purpose that allows them to find meaning in what they are doing and to 'go for it', rather than passivity and avoidance.
- **Control** is the tendency to feel and act as if one is influential rather than helpless. Interestingly, it does not seem to matter too much whether it is objective or subjective control (e.g. I am

in control of the situation, or I think myself to be in control), or even the situation is under control. This is in contrast with the 'victim attitude' of someone who feels that the centre of control lies outside them.

- **Challenge** is a disposition that sees change as an opportunity rather than a threat. It leads to attempts to transform and grow in response to new situations rather than to conserve and protect.

All three of these attributes can also be seen to relate to having a self-concept that is not dependent on external conditions of worth, but rather rests on a high degree of self-acceptance.[9] As long as I believe in my own inherent value, what is external can never truly undermine it.

Spend a few minutes considering first your own situation and job. How do you rate the commitment, control and challenge you hold? Is there any way you would like to change them? Then consider the situation of any patient of yours and see what light it might throw on either their illness or the way the medical system treats them.

Measuring your own stress requires looking at your life in both a dynamic and compassionate way, from the point of view of the pressures you are subject to and the way you react to those pressures. Some things may be unchangeable, but much may be open to modification. If we want to reduce our stress, we must take the initiative at both a personal and professional level.

References

1 Kobasa S, Maddi S and Kahn S (1982) Hardiness and health: a prospective study. *J Person Soc Psychol.* **42**: 168–77.

2 Kanner AD *et al.* (1981) Comparison of two modes of stress measurement: Daily hassles and uplifts versus major life events. *J Behav Med.* **4**: 1–39.

3 The Yately Stress Group (1993) In: *Stress Management in General Practice.* Occasional Paper 61. Royal College of General Practitioners, London.

4 Rogers C (1961) *On Becoming a Person.* Constable, London.

5 Maslow AH (1954) *Motivation and Personality.* Harper and Row, London.

6 Sackin P, Barnett M, Eastaugh A and Paxton P (1997) Peer supported learning. *Br J Gen Pract.* **Feb:** 67–8.

7 RCGP (1993) *Portfolio-based Learning in General Practice.* Occasional Paper 63. Royal College of General Practitioners, London.

8 Howie J *et al.* (1993) In *Stress Management in General Practice.* Occasional Paper 61. Royal College of General Practitioners, London, pp. 18–31.

9 Thorne B (1992) *Carl Rogers.* Sage, London.

3 Burnout

Sidha Sambandan

Stress is an inevitable part of life, but Suffering is optional.

Burnout is not unique to the medical profession or even to the caring professions. It is being increasingly observed everywhere, even in the Third World, and especially in the business sector where entrepreneurs are succumbing to the rapid pace of change.

An academic definition of burnout describes it as an interactive process experienced by an individual which depends on the perceived demands of *relentless work related stress* and the *cognitive appraisal* of the demands in the light of the *personal coping resources*.[1] The first documentation of burnout seems to have been in 1974 by Dr Herbert Freudenberger.[2]

Although burnout can occur in any age and occupation, it has been observed to be more common in younger healthcarers, between one to three years after starting a job. General practitioners (the 'gatekeepers' of primary care) are particularly vulnerable.

The term 'burnout' was initially derived from rocket science. Even when a rocket has exhausted its fuel, it continues to move forward and appears still to be useful, even though it is actually no longer functioning. Although graphically apt, the term seems to imply a stage of 'no return'. This is not so. Burnout can be reversed. However, it implies a stage where external help or facilitation (by a skilled counsellor or colleague/mentor skilled in stress management) is often needed. This return of 'equilibrium' usually takes time.

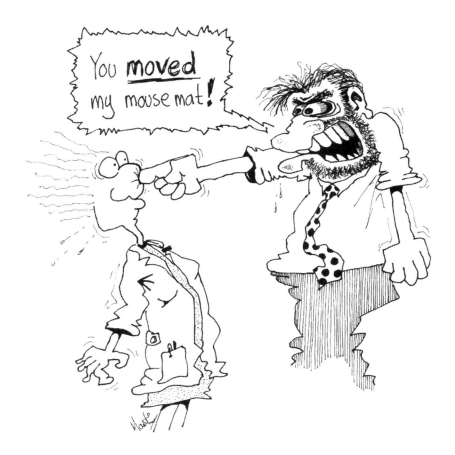

Mechanisms of burnout

Two major interacting groups of factors are involved in an individual's experience of burnout.

- **Personal factors:**
  - *Personality factors.* Includes how we handle our emotions like anger, and how positive our attitude is to the situations we experience. Persistent negative attitude increases the vulnerability to burnout.

– *Physical factors.* Physical illness or disability. The effects of chronic illness, be it mental or physical, can have an impact on the way we cope with our stressors.

– *Cultural factors.* Cultural factors are also important. This may reflect the general lifestyle of the society in which the individual lives.

– *Cognitive factors.* How we perceive and appraise an event or situation – as loss, harm, threat or challenge.[1]

– *Coping strategies.* Our personal resources[3] and strategies, which we are able to utilise to manage the stressful event, at that time.

- **Environmental factors**: we experience external stressors in our daily life, including major life events and the daily hassles of life. Other factors are workload and other loads. They are only triggers, and not the only cause of the stress syndrome. Major factors that act as stressors in the professional context are as follows:

  – *Information overload.* The rapid advance in information technology has resulted in an information explosion, accessible by anybody – both patients and doctors. The globe has shrunk with the advent of electronic mail and the worldwide web. This has necessitated new skills for the medical profession – the ability to search, select and critically appraise the information. This has to be applied to practice, which is the ultimate purpose of the exercise.

  – *Rapid advances in medical technology.* These have necessitated the development of new knowledge and skills in diagnostic and therapeutic procedures, as well as making the concept of rationing much more explicit, with a risk that it could erode the doctor–patient relationship.

  – *Expanding workload, within shrinking financial and material resources.* Increasing consumerism has resulted in both increasing demands and expectations from patients. In addition, doctors find themselves also accountable to both managers and consumers, with the attendant stresses that inevitably follow.

- *Increasing patient expectations and demands.* Patient expectations and demands have increased over the past few years. The public is better 'informed' and, in the UK, media publicity about substandard practice in a few of the NHS Trusts has resulted in the demand for greater professional regulation by the stake-holders and the public.

Burnout is the extreme form of stress syndrome. The effect of increasing stress arousal on an individual's performance can be explained by Yerkes–Dodson's Law,[4] which has been modified by Melhuish.[5] This describes how performance increases only up to a point when the pressure stimulus/stress increases in intensity. The modified graph (Figure 3.1) shows four stages. In stage A, when the stimulus is below a certain threshold, the effect is negative, due to insufficiency of the arousal to stimulate or motivate performance. I would prefer to call this phenomenon *rustout,* as opposed to stage D – at the other extreme – where relentless stress leads to burnout. Rustout is a result of *boredom,* and *lack of commitment and motivation* to perform, resulting in *apathy, lack of interest and low energy.* Stage B is where the performance increases with increasing levels of pressure – up to a limit. This is exhibited by

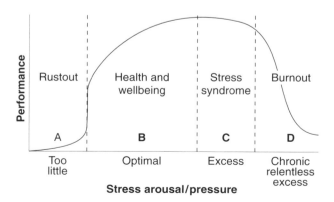

Figure 3.1 Effect of stress arousal or pressure on performance: a personal view.

an increasing sense of wellbeing and health with optimal to maximal performance. In stage C, further increase in stress or pressure results in diminished performance, with accompanying signs and symptoms of the stress syndrome. Chronic, relentless, excess of stress or pressure leads to burnout, which is stage D, where the performance declines steeply, accompanied by physical, mental and emotional exhaustion and negative attitude.

Burnout, unlike rustout, occurs in individuals who in the past have been performing optimally, if not maximally, and have been motivated to perform well. The introduction of the NHS reforms and new contract since 1990, followed by the rapid changes in the provision of care, compounded by increasing expectations from patients (subsequent to the introduction of the Patient's Charter) and the shifting of care from the hospitals to the community, have resulted in an increasing workload, information overload and time pressure. These have been instrumental in causing increasing stress and burnout amongst GPs since 1990. Similar situations are arising in other countries. The recent changes in the NHS, with the advent of PCGs, has led to further increases in the demand for GPs' time, with a significant proportion of general practitioners having to work on PCG Boards, at the expense of time spent with their patients.

Burnout is caused by many interlinked factors. Due to individual variation in coping strategies, cognitive appraisals and personalities, the same stimulus or cause may affect different doctors to different extents under the same circumstances. The following list is by no means comprehensive. Most are common to all healthcare workers.

- **Primary, personal and continued care**, and the resultant physical, mental, social and spiritual interactive demands. Being the 'gatekeeper' and the 'gateway' to other levels of care, the GP has to respond to all the demands made by patients who seek help. He or she is contractually obliged to do so 24 hours of the day. Thus, the very nature of the GP's job demands repetitive contact with people, being the first and direct care provider. Being personal, the intensity of the psychosocial interaction is high. Continuity of care demands long-term continued interaction. General practice, by its very nature, is a high-stress profession. It has been classified as a profession with high demand and high decision latitude.[6] The high demand is not necessarily perceived as stressful, as long as there is also freedom of action and autonomy in decision making. Unfortunately, the latter has been eroded with the post-1990 changes in the NHS. GPs as self-employed doctors have cherished their independence for many years. Since the advent of PCGs, operational since April 1999, there has been a political need for GPs to work more closely together to provide quality care for their population. GPs have to get accustomed to a cultural transformation from independence to interdependence. Many senior GPs find it difficult to adapt to the rapid changes, resulting in long-term sickness or early retirement. Uncertainties surrounding the neophyte PCGs have led to declining morale in most areas of the country.

- **The 'giving' role.** This is common to all healthcare workers, where the 'consumer' perceives the 'receiving' of care as a right.
- **Demands made by a specific group of patients** – 'Heartsink' patients. This is of special relevance to primary care, where a small cohort of patients is known to cause excessive demands in their interaction with the GP. They may use strategies like persistent denying, demanding and dependency, which may lead to frustrations in the GP. Some have felt that the problem is greater from the perspective of the GP who cannot cope!
- **Dealing with the chronically sick, dying and death.** This can be emotionally demanding.
- **Job monotony and lack of opportunities for personal and professional development** through career structures after becoming a principal. GPs who have taken the initiative to pursue other interests or occupations by doing 'sessions' in hospitals or by taking on other commitments, such as

education, have avoided the monotony. The increasing availability of further education, leading to Diplomas, Masters courses and Fellowship by assessment, is facilitating the professional development of primary care physicians. The chief constraints are lack of protected time, accessibility and affordability. Continuing professional development is increasingly becoming an industry, deliberated by part-time academics from a central institution far removed from the real world of full-time practitioners. Many practitioners are concerned about the further demands on time and resources that are inevitable with the implementation of structured, portfolio-based personal development plans, practice development plans and revalidation requirements that will be mandatory from 2001.

- **Inability to adapt to rapid changes.** Change is endemic in general practice, whether it be the 'New GP Contract' in 1990, the advent of PCGs in 1999, the 'Patient's Charter', fundholding, or the shift of care into the community. All these have necessitated adaptation within time constraints. From coping with change, through responding to change, GPs have to thrive on accelerating change. The recent management infiltration into primary care has imposed a sense of time pressure – to accomplish more and more within limited time scales. Research has shown that doctors experienced more stress, less job satisfaction and poorer mental health in 1990 than in 1987.[7] The exit of fundholding in 1999 and the advent of PCGs have marginalised the needs of smaller practices, especially when they are not represented on the Boards.

- **Absence of roles and boundaries.** In the context of the rapid changes in primary care, the 'job' of the GP has become seamless. Lack of a job description defining the roles, responsibilities and boundaries of care has compounded the workload, information overload and response to changes in educational and organisational needs.

- **Absence of external support systems.** External support systems include family, friends and professional colleagues and peers. Communication and rapport between partners is a powerful buffer against burnout. Closer working between practices in a PCG, if managed optimally, could help to prevent burnout in practitioners. Involvement of all the constituent practices, transparency, openness and communication are powerful anti-dotes to PCG failures, and will help to overcome the perception of threat felt by practitioners.

Symptoms and signs of burnout

1   In the early stages, the symptoms and signs of the *stress syndrome* are evident. Working longer hours (for example, when a partner is absent) or taking on more responsibilities of administrative or clinical work occurs in the early phase. The result is frustration from inability to achieve unrealistic goals. More time is spent on work, at the expense of family and social life – an important support mechanism. Coffee breaks and lunches are skipped. Often vacations are postponed or cancelled. 'Hurry and worry' escalates and sense of humour declines.

2   Physical, mental and emotional exhaustion are cardinal signs of burnout. The feeling of tiredness all the time, coupled with a persistent feeling of emptiness. Fatigue despite adequate sleep is very common in burnout. Emotional exhaustion is the end stage of emotional lability, with mood swings and a low threshold for irritability, directed at staff and patients. There is a tendency to blame others. At its extreme it could lead to depression with suicidal ideation. Physical exhaustion may lead to experience of physical illness and complaints such as muscle tension, headaches, dyspepsia, insomnia and low back pain.

3 Loss of job satisfaction and self-esteem: there are lowered feelings of personal accomplishments, leading to learned helplessness and defensive coping.
4 Negative attitude to self (hopeless and helpless feeling) and others (feeling of being hassled by patients and staff); depersonalisation, leading to the treatment of people as objects.
5 Increasing social withdrawal and isolation.
6 Self-medication begins or increases. Use of benzodiazepines, caffeinism and increased alcohol consumption are more common than substance abuse.

Burnout is an insidious process. Unless the individual has a high degree of awareness and reflects on his practice, it is difficult to detect burnout early. Often the partners or staff notice the changes. Unfortunately very few would be 'open' enough to approach the individual. Comments such as 'Are you alright?', 'You look tired', 'You look as if you need a holiday', 'You are not your usual happy self', 'You have changed', 'Calm down' are significant, especially if you hear them often from the staff and your partners, with similar remarks at home from the family or friends.

Maslach's Burnout Inventory,[8] which measures three aspects of the burnout syndrome (Figure 3.2) has been used in a number of studies of burnout in nurses and hospital doctors. There is a paucity of research into burnout in GPs. In an American study of burnout among 67 family practice residents,[9] it was noted that long hours, little time for leisure activities and social contact, and compulsive personality characteristics may contribute to moderate

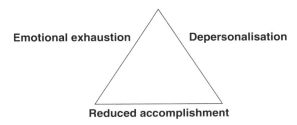

Figure 3.2   Maslach's triad of burnout.

levels of burnout. In a study done as early as 1984,[10] 87% of 156 Aberdeen GPs complained of periods of exhaustion, and 68% found their work stressful.

The following exercise will help you to recognise extreme job-related stress or burnout. A simple agree/disagree answer is adequate. The duration of the symptoms should be at least four weeks.

- When I wake up in the morning I dread the idea of going to work.
- I feel tired all the time.
- I seem to be 'behind time' and unable to catch up with the work I have to do.
- I tend to be irritable, and get angry easily with patients, partners and staff.
- I have an increasing tendency to blame others.
- I don't care about what my patients, partners or staff think of me.
- I spend less time listening to my patients during consultations.
- I tend to prescribe more.
- Increasingly, I resent the idea of visiting patients at home or advising them over the phone.
- I feel that most of my patients are very demanding and make unfair requests.
- I feel very isolated in my job and notice a sense of withdrawal from my patients, partners and staff.
- I feel I have no time for friends and family.
- Lately, I have not had the time for off-work activities such as sports or other interests.
- I have to forego my coffee breaks and lunch breaks due to the pressure of work.
- I feel very negative about general practice and its future. 'I see no light at the end of the tunnel.'
- I find it difficult to concentrate at work or at home.
- Increasingly, I feel trapped and that I have lost my autonomy and control.

- I have sleep disturbance.
- I have started taking sleeping tablets, so that I could get some sleep before another long day.
- I have a tendency to drink more coffee at work, while seeing patients.
- I have a tendency to drink more alcohol.
- I tend to have frequent colds, flu or headaches.
- Most of my consultations are either trivial or inappropriate.
- I would rather not discuss my work with my partners or colleagues.
- Tears well up in my eyes often, for no obvious reason.
- Increasingly I feel that we ought to go by our 'terms of service' when dealing with our patients.
- I have lost the enthusiasm and joy I once had for my job.
- I only do my job to earn a living.
- I hate attending practice meetings.
- I feel I am working much harder and longer, but achieving less and less.

The above inventory was designed by the author, due to the need for an easy and quick questionnaire to detect extreme stress or burnout, unlike the comprehensive Maslach Burnout Inventory. The Norwich Extreme Stress Inventory (NESI) was piloted initially on 22 doctors, and was modified to the above questionnaire of 30 questions. It has been validated subsequently against the Maslach Burnout Inventory by a psychiatrist and GP in the south of England.

If you have agreed to over 10 statements, it is very likely that you are experiencing burnout. If you have agreed to more than 20 statements, it is very likely that you are experiencing severe burnout and you need help. I have omitted many of the physical symptoms of burnout, since GPs often do not complain of physical symptoms of excessive stress, such as breathlessness, palpitations, chest pain, rapid breathing, 'butterflies in the stomach', gastrointestinal disturbances, tremors, etc. This is probably due to the 'Dr Kildare' syndrome of medical invulnerability, where doctors are not expected to fall ill and are reluctant to concede to any illness. If you have burnout and, in addition, feel depressed to the point of having recurrent suicidal ideation, you need urgent help. It is important to confide your problem to your own GP or professional friend and colleague who can help. A peer or psychologist with skills in stress management can be a great help.

The most important aspect of burnout is its prevention. The first requirement for prevention is the awareness and anticipation of burnout. Prevention could be approached from an individual level or the practice level.

Prevention of burnout

Personal strategies

The IDEAL model[11] of problem solving (Box 3.1) is an easy and useful structure to follow in the context of general practice.

Box 3.1   The IDEAL problem solver

Identify the problems
Define the problems
Explore possible strategies
Act on the strategies
Look back and evaluate the effects

Major life events

Major life events are difficult to prevent.[12] But our attitude and appraisal of these events can be changed.

Daily hassles

For the next five minutes, make a list of your daily hassles.[13] Now consider how you could avoid each hassle. For example, a GP considered the early morning traffic while driving to work a significant hassle. Exploring the options, such as listening to his favourite music in his car, taking an alternative route or leaving home 15 minutes earlier, he opted for the latter. On the days he was 'late' he took an alternative route.

Workload

Using the **IDEAL** model, the following steps may be useful.

1   Make a list of the work factors that you consider as a problem from *your perspective.*
2   List at least three different options for dealing with each problem.
3   Decide on *which* option you will take, *how* you will implement it and by *when.*
4   *Act* on your plan.
5   *Review* the progress, and *revise* your plan if needed.

How would you use the above model to consider the following?

* Increasing paperwork in the practice.
* Out-of-hours work, including night visits.
* Telephone interruptions during consultations.
* Emergency appointments.
* Reduced budget for prescribing.

Work stress could be reduced, if not avoided, by paying attention to the following issues.

Time management

This is the single most important factor to consider. How you spend the 24 hours of the day, especially the time you spend in non-work activities and the proportion of time spent on the family, also has a bearing on the way you face your work time. According to the experience of stress management workshops, the most common stressor in this area was found to be dealing with the daily paperwork that practitioners receive. An effective strategy is to use the four Ds of time management to deal with paperwork. Every time you take up a written communication in your hands, decide very quickly what you are going to do with it, after scanning the contents. You could:

- **Dump** it, especially the junk mail that manages to arrive in the tray.
- **Delegate** it. If someone else in the team could deal with it effectively, it is far better to delegate it to that individual.
- **Delay** it. If the task is not urgent, you could decide to delay it by putting it into a 'pending' tray. But, keep it to a minimum. Remember, procrastination is the thief of time!
- **Do** it. Deal with it then and there. If it is important and urgent, try to deal with it immediately. There is golden rule of picking up a communication only once! Remember, the time to do something is *now*!

Improving communication skills

This includes interpersonal skills, managing teams, leadership skills and negotiating skills. This is especially important in the context of the primary healthcare teams and PCGs. Communication includes consultation skills, telephone communication skills, interpersonal communication with others and also writing skills. Neurolinguistic programming (NLP) is a very useful tool for enhancing communication skills, especially in the non-verbal dimension of communication.

Other important issues

- Delegation of tasks to appropriate staff.
- Sharing and discussing difficult patients with partners or colleagues (e.g. young practitioners groups). Regular partnership and practice meetings allow protected time for discussion.

- Ensuring that you take mini-breaks – for coffee or doing something totally different.
- Taking lunch breaks – away from the practice premises.
- Avoid taking your work home, and bringing your home problems to work.
- Set realistic goals. Never bite off more than you can chew.

Managing work effectively does not mean that you are doing it efficiently. *Doing things right is more important than doing the right thing!*

Personality factors

Research has shown that type A personalities[14] tend to be vulnerable to stress-related problems, including ischaemic heart disease (IHD). Type A individuals tend to be aggressive and hostile; they strive for achievement, in haste – a persistent sense of time urgency. Of these traits, hostility and aggressiveness were found to have a definite correlation with IHD. It is impossible to change all the traits that make up your personality. But hostility can be sublimated to hardiness, which seems to be cardioprotective. Redford Williams[15] suggested 12 ways in which one could control anger, aggressiveness and hostility – based on our ability to develop more trust in others. These include reducing your cynical mistrust of others' motives, reducing the frequency and intensity of your emotional reactions (keeping a 'hostility log', acknowledging your problem and thought stopping), reasoning with yourself, taking the role of the other person, learning to laugh at yourself, practising trust, learning to be assertive and practising forgiveness.

Hardiness[16] is a personality style characterised by three Cs – a sense of **commitment**, **control** and a perception of problems as **challenges** rather than threats. I would add two other Cs – being **composed** (a reflection of grace and grit) and **competence**. Composure and competence lead to confidence.

Developing the traits of a trusting heart and hardiness may prevent stress-related illnesses and burnout.

Physical factors

Paying attention to lifestyle, especially factors such as diet, exercise, not smoking, moderation in alcohol consumption, taking medication regularly – if one is on long-term medication (e.g. antihypertensives) – and avoiding being overweight.

Coping resources and strategies

Conscious positivism and social support systems are the most important.

Conscious positivism

This is an attitude and a philosophy. Looking at a glass partly filled with water, the negativist is concerned that it is half empty, while the positivist considers it half full! A positivist is an optimist who transforms a threat into opportunities and weakness into strengths. The attitude of 'unconditional positive regard' for others, as advocated by Carl Rogers, is excellent prophylaxis against stress and burnout. Remember, nothing is good or bad – but thinking makes it so.

Social support

How much support do you get from your family, friends and peers? Doctors who have a wide network of friends and professional colleagues who meet frequently have the opportunity to share their problems, and get information, advice, feedback and emotional support. In an unpublished survey by the author on GP stresses prior to and after the advent of an out-of-hours co-operative, doctors who scored over 12 before the co-operative reduced their score to under 5 after the advent of the co-operative. However, a larger, more recent study[17] has shown that although the out-of-hours service has reduced stress levels regarding particular stressors, other stressors, such as increasing patient demands, have gained importance, as a result of the recent changes in the NHS.

This illustrates the dynamic nature of stressors and stresses perceived by individuals and organisations. The current trends in small group learning provide the appropriate setting for social support. Four types of social support have been described.[18]

1 *Emotional*: family and friends are important resources for social support.
2 *Appraisal*: formative appraisal is a useful way of getting social support from peers.
3 *Informational*: this form of support can be provided by others in the work environment or outside the work setting.
4 *Instrumental*: this form of help can be provided by peers or others. For example, if you are searching for an important piece of information or reference, and you get frustrated in not being able to solve the problem, the local library staff may be able to find the necessary information.

Other coping strategies

These can include relaxation exercises, hypnosis, autogenic training, breathing exercises, yoga and meditation, massage and physical exercise. Mini-breaks at work, long weekend breaks and vacations are buffers against burnout.

Practice strategies

The practice as an organisation could have policies and programmes to reduce staff stress, by involving the whole primary care team in stress programmes. Involving staff in decisions, regular practice meetings, counselling staff, reducing role ambiguity, and staff social events can help to prevent or reduce stress and burnout.

General practitioners and other healthcare workers are particularly vulnerable to burnout. Early awareness, acknowledgement of the problem and seeking help can prevent a GP from being burned out. It is others who detect it early in you. Having a good, socially supportive network of friends and peers helps one to recognise self-burnout and early burnout in others.

The following golden rules of **burnout** prevention will help:

Belief in yourself. (Remember, if you think you can or if you think you can't – either way you are right!)

Unconditional positive regard for others. (Remember, you must trust others before others trust you!)

Regular social support and exercise. (Remember, different folks need different strokes!)

Never losing your sense of humour. (Remember, laughter is the best medicine. You use four muscles to laugh and 44 muscles to frown!)

Outings – breaks and vacations. (Remember, all work and no play, makes Jack a dull boy!)

Understand and develop hardiness. (Remember, repeat the mantra 'I don't give a damn' in your mind while smiling when you experience situational stress!)

Time management. (Remember, man says time passes; time says man passes!)

References

1 Lazarus RS and Folkman S (1984) *Stress, Appraisal and Coping.* Springer, New York.

2 Freudenberger HJ (1974) Staff burnout. *J Soc Iss.* **30** (1): 159–65.

3 Hobfoll SE (1989) Conservation of resources: A new attempt at conceptualising stress. *Am Psychol.* **44**: 513–24.

4 Yerkes RM and Dodson JD (1908) The relation of strength of stimulus to rapidity of habit-formation. *J Comp Neurol Psychol.* **18**: 459–82.

5 Melhuish A (1978) *Executive Health.* Business Books, London.

6 Karasek RA Jr (1979) Job demands, job decision latitude and mental strain: implication for job re-design. *Admin Sci Quart.* **24**: 285–308.

7 Sutherland VJ and Cooper CL (1992) Job stress, satisfaction and mental health among GPs before and after introduction of the new contract. *BMJ.* **304**: 1545–8.

8 Maslach C (1982) Burnout: a social psychological analysis. In: GS Sanders and J Suls (eds) *Social Psychology of Health and Illness.* Erlbaum, Hillsdale, NJ, pp. 227–54.

9 Lemkau JP, Purdy RR, Rafferty JP and Rudisill JR (1988) Correlates of burnout among family practice residents. *J Med Educ.* **63** (9): 682–91.

10 Morrice JKW (1984) Job stress and burnout. *Br J Psychiat Bull.* **March**: 45.

11 Bransford JD and Stein BS (1984) The ideal problem solver. WH Freeman, New York.

12 Holmes TH and Rahe RH (1967) The social readjustment rating scale. *J Psychosom Res.* **11**: 213–18.

13 Kanner AD *et al.* (1981) Comparison of two modes of stress management: daily hassles and uplifts versus major life events. *J Behav Med.* **4**: 1–39.

14 Friedman M and Rosenman R (1974) *Type A Behaviour and Your Heart.* Knopf, New York.

15 Williams RB (1989) *The Trusting Heart: Great news about Type A behaviour.* Random House, New York.

16 Maddi S (1989) *Theories of Personality* (5e). Dorsey, Homewood, IL.

17 Mudge K and Braidwood L (1999) Out-of-hours service reduces stress levels in general practitioners. *J Clin Govern.* **7**: 48–51.

18 House JS (1981) *Work, Stress and Social Support.* Addison Wesley, Reading, MA.

4 Women and stress

Kate Wishart

The majority of women today work. Theoretically, women have the same educational and employment opportunities as men. Women make up over half of medical school intakes, but they are very much in the minority in most specialties. General practice would seem to offer an ideal setting for combining work and family, but even here men outnumber women. However, this is changing. Fifty-six per cent of all GP registrars are now women, and the proportion of female general practitioners rose by 10% between 1985 and 1995, to 31%.[1]

Many of the reasons that women have particular problems in general practice stem from society's expectations of women. This was especially true in the past, but is still partly so today. The traditional womanly virtues include many of the attributes valued highly in the caring professions. These are warmth, sensitivity, the ability to listen and empathise, kindness and the instinct to nurture. However, the traits that can protect against the effects of stress are seen as mainly male attributes. These include assertiveness, ambition, efficiency, competence and professionalism. Women GPs must therefore acquire some of these skills without losing their caring ones. The danger is that in becoming more business-like they may be perceived as more 'masculine' and even as a threat.

Women GPs face special problems in three areas of their lives: at work, at home and at the work–home interface. All of these can cause stress and each has different aspects.

The practice

Sadly, there is still discrimination against women. First, let us look at the problem of getting a partnership. Many women are tied to an area because of their husband's job. This leaves them with weaker bargaining power and there is potential for exploitation of a woman who has little choice of practice area if she wants to work. A practice wanting a partner may have false expectations. Partners may assume that a woman would want part-time work at least until her family has grown up. They might rule out a woman candidate for a full-time post at the short-listing stage, especially if she is married and of childbearing age. When interviewing women, questions about plans for having children and arrangements for child-care are still asked, despite discrimination on such grounds being illegal. What woman would refuse to answer such questions at the risk of losing her chance of the job? A woman may also be wrongly perceived as less likely to want to buy into the practice.

Once a partner, a woman GP may come up against more false expectations. She may find it difficult to agree the form of a partnership agreement. Clauses she might have to fight for include those on maternity leave, buying a share of the buildings and the possibility of changing her commitment should the partnership change. Indeed, many women do not get the chance of signing a partnership agreement.

Maternity leave may be regarded as a threat, despite arrangements for reimbursement of locum fees, as these seldom cover the actual cost of a replacement. Other partners see it as disruptive and, I suspect, may feel slightly envious of the opportunity of having 3 months out of the practice. Male partners may assume that a woman GP will not be interested in the business side of the practice and exclude her from certain of the administrative decisions. When business meetings are held in the evenings, a woman may find it more difficult to attend. This makes her involvement in such decision making more difficult and male partners may question her commitment and interest.

Being stereotyped at work

In the day-to-day work of the practice, a female GP may find herself being stereotyped. She might be expected to take on most of the 'women's problems' of the practice. These would include antenatal care, gynaecology, family planning and many psychological problems in women patients. Her interests, however, might lie in a completely different direction. Interestingly, Graffy[2] found that the choice of a woman doctor had more to do with general preference than the specific problem the patient was presenting. However, a survey conducted in 1996 found that women GPs were much more likely to be responsible for the health of women patients, whereas the men GPs tended to be more involved with minor surgery and computers.[3]

Because of the feminine attributes mentioned above, women GPs tend to have a more patient-centred approach to the consultation. A study of stress in GPs practising in Lothian showed that high stress scores were more strongly associated with a patient-centred approach than a non-patient-centred approach.[4] However, patient-centred consulting styles are also associated with greater job satisfaction. Patient-centred consultations tend to be longer and this makes running late more likely. This is, in itself, a potent cause of stress.

Another traditional caring trait is difficulty in saying 'no'. Women, of course, do not have a monopoly in this, but their upbringing is more likely to have made it harder for them to refuse to help. Thus they may be regarded both by patients and by reception staff as a 'soft touch'. This can add to their workload and therefore to their stress.

Practice reception and administration staff are usually women. Staff may treat a female GP differently to a male GP, especially in

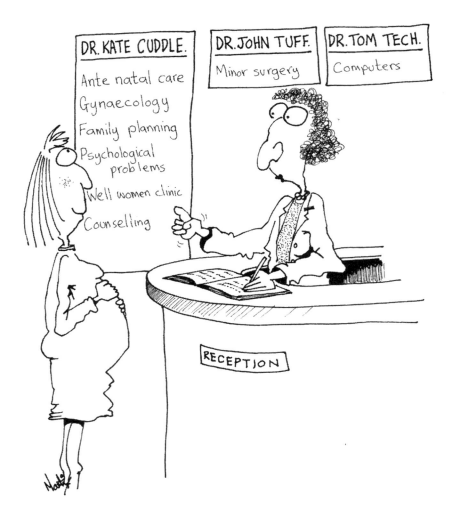

respect of the small comforts. Where they will gladly make tea for and pamper their male employer (especially if he is young), they may not take kindly to a woman GP who expects the same treatment. This is rather like the way male junior housemen are mothered by their ward nurses, while the female houseman has to do all her own dirty work.

Patients can be discriminatory too. All GPs are at risk of sexual harassment and violence, but a woman may be perceived as an easier target than a man. And it may be that someone who feels the need to show aggression to his or her doctor would choose a woman GP, if possible, for maximum effect with minimum risk. General practice journals are full of stories about the violence offered to GPs. This publicity is likely to increase the fears of women GPs and thus increase their stress, especially when out on visits.

The home

'Home is the girl's prison and the woman's workhouse.' Society has moved on since George Bernard Shaw wrote those words, but they still have an element of truth. Women still bear the brunt of the responsibility for running the home and caring for the children.

Most working women have two jobs, one paid and one unpaid. The fact that the homemaker's role is an unpaid one communicates to the woman's subconscious that housework is not important and therefore not of the same value as her paid job. Moreover, the never-ending nature of 'women's work' in the home often precludes a woman from ever feeling that she has achieved a measurable and worthwhile result. Of course, many husbands help their wives with the household chores and with the care of their children, but all too often their help is seen as a bonus, rather than a matter of responsibility. Women who work outside the home feel just as tired and stressed as do men when they come in from work. A working wife and mother must find the time and energy to shop, cook, clean, wash and iron clothes as well as chauffeur her children to their sports matches, supervise homework and music practice and comfort her husband when he has had a hard day at work. As a result she is often too tired to spend time on those things that protect against the effects of stress. We all need time for leisure activities, quiet reflection, relaxation and exercise. It is also important to find time for relationships and for maintaining a network of friends.

Coping with motherhood and work?

Mothers and wives are perceived as the caring, nurturing part of the family. Mum is usually the person to whom the toddler will go for comfort when he falls over and the one who always knows what to do for Granny's sore knee. So a female GP cannot put off her caring role when she gets home. She must still be a listener and show interest in all her family tells her, however she is feeling. All GPs find it difficult to fulfil the expectations of their families and friends when someone is ill. I know how resentful male colleagues feel, and how unsympathetically they react if one of the family becomes ill. How much harder for a GP mother to unravel the resentment from the instinct to care for her family.

Providing child-care is fraught with worry for a working mother. Nannies are expensive and good ones difficult to come by. They often require living accommodation and a car, and their wages are twice taxed, once in their name and once in their employer's name. Childminders are an acceptable alternative but one that takes the child away from home, possibly for long hours. Nurseries are scarce, particularly in rural areas, and are again expensive, so the working mother must earn sufficient to make it worth her while to work at all. Added to all this are the pressures, real or perceived, subtle or blatant, from family and friends who do not approve of working mothers. A community nursing sister I know felt irritated when a friend commented, 'Your poor husband, I often wonder if he gets a meal in the middle of the day!' What made her really cross was that it left her faintly worried about him too, despite the fact that she knows he is perfectly capable of getting a meal for himself. Children join in with this game too; 'Why didn't you come to my sports day, Mummy? All the other mummies were there'. And 'You never take us swimming'. It all adds up to a woman believing that she should feel guilty about working, and many of us end up feeling exceedingly guilty, usually without good reason. In addition, when the children are old enough to look after themselves, women often find themselves responsible for the care of an elderly relative.

Another problem almost always faced by the woman in a family, is what happens when either the nanny, the childminder or one of the children is ill? Does she stay at home, and how will her partners view it if she does? Should her husband stay at home? The 1996 survey found that only 2% of women GPs said that their partner would do so, whereas 66% of male GPs thought that their partner would look after the children.[3] So the expectation is that the mother will be the main carer in this situation. This all adds to the stress for the GP mother, whose guilt is then triggered by the thought of letting her colleagues down.

The work–home interface

Being on call used to be one of the prime stressors for GPs.[5] Thankfully, for most of us this situation has been relieved by the formation of co-operatives and deputising services for night and weekend cover. On-call duties are now usually done in dedicated centres as shifts, thus disrupting home life much less than in the days of 24-hour duties. The stress and fear of night visits for women is also reduced as most of these co-operatives employ drivers, with radio or telephone contact to the co-op centre. However, there are still some women doing on-call duties from home and trying to juggle calls and home visits with preparing meals and laundry duties.

Solutions

Tension arises from the differences between what we believe and the reality. For instance, a woman who believes that a good mother stays at home with her children will feel guilty and therefore stressed if she goes out to work. Women must therefore either change their beliefs or change the reality. A woman GP must first learn to believe herself the equal of a male GP. She must build up her self-esteem as a working woman who has much to offer. She must remind herself daily of those qualities that make her so well suited to her profession. Once she can believe these things about herself, the rest is straightforward. It involves learning those skills that make life easier and release time for relaxation, exercise and leisure. These skills will be of value in the home as well as at work and can be applied anywhere.

A woman GP must have a clear idea of what is important to her. Does she want a true partnership or would she be happier as a salaried assistant? Is she prepared to sacrifice income for convenient hours, and if so, to what extent? It is so much easier to get what you want if you can ask for it clearly and make a good case for it. Therefore, assertiveness is essential. It allows one to state one's needs and wants clearly and reasonably and helps one to persevere until they are achieved. It will stop others being patronising and will feed a blossoming self-esteem. Organisation is also vital. Time management skills are well worth the study, and being well prepared for meetings is a great help in achieving one's objectives.

It is also important to know the true monetary value of one's time. Knowing that you can earn £60 in an hour filling in medical reports will make you feel better about paying someone much less to do the cleaning and ironing, and you will gain time for other things into the bargain. Learning to delegate will repay time and trouble. Make a rota for housework, washing and ironing, and publish it with confidence. Don't let the family get away with delegating it back. When asking others to do things, be specific and make sure they understand exactly what you want them to do.

Looking after yourself is also important. Regular exercise, formal relaxation and quiet time, together with healthy eating habits, all protect against the effects of stress, as well as leaving one fitter and healthier. Finally, having and maintaining a close and confiding relationship with a partner or friend will be a great support when things get tough.[6]

Summary

The particular problems for women in general practice stem partly from society's expectations of them. Other pressures result from the need to balance the working role with that of the wife and mother at home. Women GPs who feel stressed by these conflicts can improve their lifestyles and their coping ability by acquiring new skills.

References

1 Royal College of General Practitioners (1998) *Women General Practitioners.* RCGP Information Sheet No. 14, October. RCGP, London.

2 Graffy J (1990) Patient choice in a practice with men and women. *Gen Pract.* **40** (330): 13–15.

3 Chambers R and Campbell I (1996) Gender differences in general practitioners at work. *Br J Gen Pract.* **46**: 291–3.

4 Howie J, Porter M and Heaney D (1993) General practitioners, work and stress. In: *Stress Management in General Practice.* Occasional Paper 61. Royal College of General Practitioners, London.

5 Royal College of General Practitioners (1998) *Stress and General Practice.* RCGP Information Sheet No. 22, October. RCGP, London.

6 Rout U and Rout JK (1993) *Stress and General Practitioners.* Kluwer Academic Press, London.

5 The stresses of clinical medicine

Simon Brown

Perhaps you are thinking that this is the bit that we can all do – the 'nuts and bolts' clinical doctoring part of medicine. We all know how stressful the politics of a changing health service has been and is likely to continue to be. We all face a daunting uphill struggle against piles of paper, the clock, increasingly demanding patients, complaints, managing our practices and doing more and more for less – just to name but a few of our demons. But the clinical medicine is surely the enjoyable bit where our training takes over and tells us what to do, even in a crisis. After all we are doctors, aren't we?

Of course, the reality of day-to-day clinical practice is very different. Despite the training we have already received, there is a disparity between what we achieve and what is expected of us. This gap between supply and demand, both physical and psychological, is an inevitable part of life, let alone work in today's primary care. This is the stuff of stress, the lynchpin of potential unhappiness unless we are able to understand and resolve the difference for ourselves as people, GPs and the profession as a whole. This is an important process, not simply a political justification of our finite limits as individuals or the appropriate core tasks of GPs. If we get it right, we may just feel contentment in a job well done.

I am going to take a bet with you now that the thing that stresses you most is different from my worst nightmare? Recently in my practice we were looking at working patterns and each of the doctors was given the opportunity to identify the most stressful situation that they most commonly encountered. For some this was a long list of telephone calls to be squeezed in before going out to do visits. But for another doctor hearing the reception staff saying to patients that we had no more available appointments drove him to walk out of earshot. We know that a particular stress will not hold the same importance for everybody and the coping strategies they employ will be very different. So there is a small risk that as you read the rest of this chapter the elements of stress arising from practising clinical medicine and the solutions I offer will miss your biggest stressor or your best solution. I hope that there are elements both of problems and answers that ring true for you as well.

Why might clinical medicine be stressful? I have tried to identify some of the elements of stress under headings as follows.

The omniscient psychic

When was the last time you made a real howler, a blindingly daft mistake, the sort of thing that as you think of it now your pulse starts to race and you begin to blush at the very recollection? Perhaps you can't think of anything. In that case you really are the superhuman sort of doctor that I wish I was. Alternatively, you may simply be adept at banishing such negative images to the depths of your subconsciousness. If you are of the amnesic, repressing type, then good luck to you. In fact, most doctors seem to carry a fair collection of error-laden baggage!

We know that a dispositional tendency to self-blame can be detected very early in our medical careers and correlates with our perceived stress levels later in our lives when we are working as doctors.[1] This feature of many of our personalities is exacerbated by the profession and our patients. Early on at medical school we are raised in an atmosphere of criticism and humiliation. I have spoken to many medical students who assure me that this is still the case. If we do not already have this trait, clinical school training encourages a very negative view of errors in judgement. You must remember the so-called 'teaching rounds', when feedback would be centred on the causes of clubbing, for example, that you had forgotten rather than those that you had actually remembered. This tendency to negative feedback continues into our working lives. However, patients exalt us to the position of omniscient beings. One of my patients recently left my room after a particularly complicated consultation saying 'I do trust you doctor!' This is perhaps warming and charming, but leaves 10% of me wanting to rush after her shouting 'I am fallible, I am human, take some responsibility for yourself!' At the same time, patients, the public and government give largely negative feedback about the service we provide. You may well have received one or more complaints yourself and these may feel entirely unjustified from your point of view. The last one I had, as the complainant later admitted, was entirely due to dissatisfaction with events at the hospital. He couldn't resist 'grapeshotting' the whole service he had received. It would be easy to believe many of the negative views presented if we failed to acknowledge the shift of our society to pick holes in most things!

Now I am not suggesting a slapdash, no-care approach to what we do. I am not suggesting that we, as individuals or as a profession, accept low standards or incompetent care, rather that we allow ourselves to believe in a positive view of ourselves and what we achieve. When was the last time someone said to you 'Hey, you did a great job!' Did you believe it, or did you discount their positive feedback either as invalid or undeserved? I place tremendous value on the thank-you letters I receive from patients and their relatives, and have a small collection that I use as a tool to reaffirm my own value when things are less good. Keep these letters and try to believe them. Try to accept compliments from patients or colleagues. Try to be encouraging and non-critical of your partners or other doctors. And the next time you make a mistake try to say 'Oops! I'm human!'

Three-dimensional chess played in the dark

Think back to your last working day. How many clinical decisions did you make? How many of those were based on a full history, examination, investigation and treatment based on the latest evidence or guideline? Perhaps you are more organised than I am, for many of my decisions are made on the much shakier ground of probability and a continuum of 'doing no harm'. When I was a house officer I would tick all the boxes on the laboratory request form for each patient arriving as an emergency in the hospital. This assured that on the subsequent ward round I had 100% sensitivity and the relevant numbers were always to hand. Clearly, we are unable to do this with respect to all investigations and, fortunately, most of us learn specificity in ordering only essential investigations. Apart from bankrupting the health service, it may be impracticable to investigate our patients extensively. My patients face a 30 mile round trip if I want them to have a chest X-ray.

So, many of us base our clinical decisions on the likelihood of disease and use methods of hypotheses and deduction to explore outcomes for that patient. In the same way that people react differently to various stressors, we vary as doctors in our comfort in tolerating such uncertainty. One of my recent registrars arrived in the practice with considerable hospital experience under his belt and tried to order extensive and complicated investigations. This caused much anxiety and inconvenience for patients, but he felt justified in 'doing the best for my patient'. He was able very slowly to shift to a style of consulting that allowed him to share his uncertainties with patients.

Our patients expect us to be certain. Clearly there are levels of uncertainty from 'I'm not sure if you have cancer' to 'I'm uncertain if you really need an antibiotic', that vary from unacceptable for all to the very stuff of general practice. But a lot of decision making is much more subtle, the sifting of serious early disease from the symptom-ridden contacts we have with patients. We are unlikely to get this process right every busy day in a professional lifetime.

Every second counts

A few years ago I persuaded my partners to equip the surgery with a defibrillator and other emergency equipment. Despite this, everyone doubted we would use it. Then one of our patients attending the surgery for a blood test had a full-blown cardiac arrest in the middle of the waiting room.

In theory this sort of thing might happen at any time. In practice, events like this are uncommon, but nevertheless we are expected to know what to do and, in medico-legal terms, to get it right. I am fortunate in holding a clinical assistantship in anaesthetics. But for many doctors the last cardiac arrest they attended will have been many years ago, perhaps in hospital days.

Retaining practical skills, such as airway management, and knowing protocols well enough to apply them without hesitation for events that happen infrequently is asking a lot of anyone. This is almost impossible without regular training. At least familiarity with emergency equipment and how to use it may make these inherently stressful situations less so. We know from studies of psychological distress in hospital doctors working in emergency situations that stress levels are inversely related to confidence in carrying out a range of clinical tasks.[2] Perhaps we need to allow ourselves a certain amount of rehearsal for the infrequent emergency situations, so at least we are better prepared when every second really does influence outcome.

Avoiding the evidence

Evidence-based medicine has become almost clichéd of late. One could argue that we do indeed practise at an evidence-based level, but that much of the 'evidence' is anecdotal and a million miles from the randomised controlled trial. This does not make it invalid evidence. At the same time, we are urged to apply guidelines to clinical care which purport to be 'evidence-based'. Cholesterol levels, blood pressures and HbA_{1c}s, to name but a few, have lower target values than ever before for the optimal management of our patients. The goals are getting harder to attain. At best, these things will certainly increase our workload. At worst, they themselves become stressors, gaps between our perception of what we have achieved and what needs to be done. Of course, these changes don't happen overnight. Every preventative intervention costs in time, effort and money. I am not suggesting we should be complacent in a situation when we might improve outcomes for our patients. At the same time, the focus is on what has not been done. The hitherto excellent chronic care is taken for granted and swept away by the latest recommendation. Perhaps we should spend a little time remembering what we have achieved for our patients so far.

Just when you thought you'd got it covered

A medical student who visited my practice recently remarked on the variety of things we had seen together in morning surgery. For her the unpredictability of whatever was coming next threw her into confusion as she swapped from one hospital-learned specialty to another. As GPs we are used to doing these acrobatics between clinical areas, let alone all the other things we deal with during a typical day. At best this is a challenge, but becomes a potential stressor, especially on those days when all the complex and time-consuming things cluster together. Do you remember the last time you wished that the next patient would bring a simple sore throat? We spend much of our time waiting for things to happen to our patients rather than being able to plan their care or our working days. At the other extreme, some GPs become stressed at the apparent lack of interest in much of the medicine they see, so missing the complexities of the interaction we have with patients as people.

Small wonder we become stressed with this catalogue of public expectations, emergency situations and unpredictable demand that we can simply only react to. On the other hand, look at all the things that you manage to cope with every day. Please allow yourself a little positive feedback. Remember, you're doing a great job, or to put it another way, you are doing a fantastic job well!

References

1 Firth-Cozens J (1997) Predicting stress in general practitioners: 10 year follow up postal survey. *BMJ*. **315**: 34–5.

2 Williams S, Dale J, Glucksman E *et al.* (1997) Senior house officers' work related stressors, psychological distress, and confidence in performing clinical tasks in accident and emergency: a questionnaire study. *BMJ*. **314**: 713.

Further reading

Von Oncuil J (1996) ABC of work related disorders: Stress at work. *BMJ*. **313**: 745–8.

6 Patients who make the doctor depressed

Paul Sackin

Case history 1

Peter is in his 40s. He has cared for his wife for the past 20 years as she has gradually gone downhill with multiple sclerosis. Now she is not only grossly physically disabled but she is also aggressive and somewhat demented. Peter used to cope well with looking after Janet in addition to his full-time job and he found the time for various hobbies and sports as well. He rarely came near the surgery. Now everything has gone wrong. He gets shoulder pain and sciatica as soon as he touches a badminton racquet, he has no motivation for work, he has difficulty organising care for Janet and he feels anxious and depressed all the time. Antidepressant medication, not surprisingly, has made no difference. He found talking to the practice counsellor of little help and he defaulted from attending. The GP sees him regularly just to listen to his woes and to try to find ways of helping. At the end of each session the doctor feels almost as miserable as Peter.

We can all recognise patients like Peter as one type of patient who can make the doctor depressed. It is very easy for depression to diffuse gently from patient to doctor, so that the patient loses some, while the doctor gains it. Perhaps it is not surprising that the doctor, as Balint[1] pointed out, is the most potent psychotropic drug of all. Nor is it surprising that GPs often feel distressed. Arguably it is an essential part of our role to absorb our patients' emotions. How to deal with these emotions when we *have* absorbed them is the subject of most of this book.

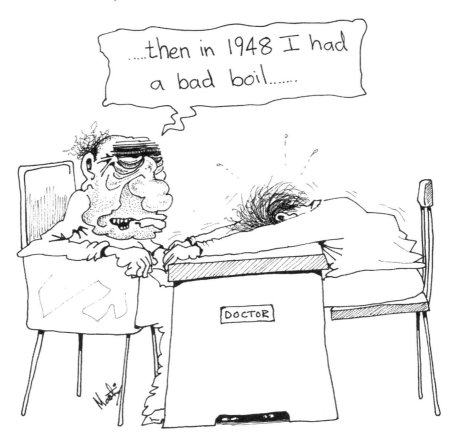

Now another type of patient, of whom each practice seems to have at least one:

Case history 2

Jean has attended the surgery an average of once or twice a week for about the past 20 years (at least 1000 consultations). Her list of organic conditions, including two major cancers, easily fills the computer screen. She is almost always pleasant and apologetic but nevertheless brings at least three problems to each consultation, often with a request for a referral or for other outside help thrown in. The slightest hint that she may be just a mite demanding leads to tears and a reminder of how she has coped with the enucleation of an eye, a total cystectomy and an impossible husband. In retrospect, there was an appalling delay before her bladder cancer was diagnosed – she had microscopic haematuria for months. Fourteen years later her GPs (fortunately she does not always see the same partner) are again feeling remorse at the delay in diagnosis of yet another cancer, but also they cannot help admiring her courage in the face of a poor prognosis honestly shared with her.

In short, overwhelming problems for both patient and doctor.

These two examples are perhaps rather extreme but they highlight a range of negative feelings that patients may incite in their doctors. 'Depression' is a useful generic word to describe these feelings, but it is really an oversimplification. The feelings engendered by these patients may well also include anxiety, anger, loss of control and frustration. These feelings may often reflect similar, though perhaps hidden, feelings in the patient. With patients such as Peter the causes of the feelings seem readily apparent, but all rational solutions to the problem upset the emotional status quo and are therefore too frightening to contemplate. With patients such as Jean there are probably fundamental problems in early life which are too painful to go near, and even the smallest attempt to look beneath the surface leads to heavy defence mechanisms being brought into play.

Less extreme types of patient can also give rise to uneasy feelings in the doctor. These feelings need to be heeded. They may give an important clue to the patient's state of mind.

Case history 3

Mr A was an accountant who moved out of London with his wife on his retirement. He managed to find various small jobs but greatly missed his work and was unable to settle in the country. He attended the surgery regularly and was clearly depressed but not unduly so. Nevertheless when his GP attended a Balint weekend, Mr A was the patient whom he decided to present because uneasy feelings about him kept coming to mind. The group discussion highlighted Mr A's feelings of emptiness and despair. Shortly afterwards, despite specialist psychiatric help, Mr A drowned himself. His GP felt very sad when this happened but both he and Mrs A felt that everything possible had been done to prevent the unhappy outcome.

Nowadays we are very aware of how common depression is and how often it can be treated, if only it is diagnosed. The doctor's feelings can be the main clue to the diagnosis. Formal psychiatric history taking is neither practicable nor usually helpful in general practice. GPs vary greatly in their ability to be in touch with their own and their patients' feelings. This may well explain much of the large variability in the prevalence of depression found in different surveys.

It may not just be the patient's emotional life that gives rise to negative feelings in the doctor. Often patients can remind doctors, consciously or otherwise, of their own unresolved psychological difficulties – from which nobody is exempt!

Case history 4

At a case discussion session a GP registrar presented a 72-year-old man who had suffered a myocardial infarction. The registrar seemed particularly anxious about the case.

During the discussion it transpired that her father was also 72 and that there were concerns about his health. Bringing this issue (and others) to consciousness seemed greatly to help the doctor's understanding and visibly relieve her anxiety.

Obviously not all our 'blocks' as GPs are as simple as that. Anyone with experience of a Balint group will know that individual participants often present the same type of difficult case – difficult to *them* because of their particular psychological make-up. Gaining insight into this is an immensely rewarding, if sometimes painful, experience. A group of us have been meeting as a Balint group to investigate some of the personal factors which make some patients particularly difficult for us to cope with. We have found that when we are in difficulty with these patients we may behave defensively and thus not be in the best position to deal with the patient appropriately. Given that we are unlikely to be a unique group of GPs, we thought it might be useful to describe our experiences in a book.[2] In the book we make some suggestions as to how to recognise and attempt to modify this unconscious defensive behaviour. I hope you will read this book but, even if you don't, perhaps you will agree that patients can arouse strong feelings in their doctors. These feelings are often suppressed and may there-fore come out later in uncomfortable or even inappropriate ways. I have no doubt that this is a cause of much stress for GPs. The traditional image of the doctor as an authority figure immune from the 'weakness' of human feelings hardly helps.

Being more aware of the feelings engendered by our patients is the first step in dealing with this important source of stress. Could I suggest you try a simple exercise to increase your awareness of your emotional response to patients? During your next consulting session write down a few words after each patient leaves about how they made you feel. Then find a colleague with whom to discuss your findings. The process of considering and sharing one's feelings should be an integral part of day-to-day general practice. Roger Neighbour aptly calls it 'housekeeping'.[3] Unfortunately, as we all know, it is often not possible to do the housekeeping when it is required:

Case history 5

A man in his 50s had a long and extremely distressing terminal illness. His GP found visiting him and his family very stressful anyway, but it was particularly difficult when she had to rush straight on to a busy antenatal clinic without any time to 'change gear'. She found support from the surgery staff was of great value, but it was rarely possible for this to be given at the time.

The next step after increasing your awareness of your feelings is to try to use them therapeutically. This is the whole basis of the approach to general practice pioneered in the seminars run by Michael Balint. Sometimes a simple, instinctive approach can work well:

Case history 6

A woman with a rather histrionic, depressive illness was admitted to a psychiatric unit. As the time came for her discharge the SHO planned to meet her husband, a high-ranking army officer, to discuss her future care. He was an extremely quiet man who had previously made it known to the hospital staff that he was finding his wife impossible to cope with and that several members of his family had dealt with stressful situations by committing suicide. At the appointed time, instead of just Mr X, the SHO was faced with Mrs X and two of their lively 20 or so-year-old children as well. The doctor felt overwhelmed by this family and, without thinking, said so. This led to a major family row over why the 'uninvited' family members had turned up. The SHO was able to 'referee' this row and help all the members of the family gain some insight into their behaviour. The session appeared to be the turning point in Mrs X's illness.

Such a direct approach as this needs to be used with care. Telling patients that they make you feel frustrated, angry or whatever, may merely antagonise them if not done sensitively. It is likely to be more successful to speculate back to patients on how you think *they* may be feeling. Your judgement about these feelings is likely to be based on how the patient makes *you* feel.

Such feedback to patients is really a simple form of psychotherapy. It can often be remarkably effective even in the context of the short GP appointment. There is an excellent example in the book *Six Minutes for the Patient*:[4]

Case history 7

A middle-aged single woman comes to the GP complaining of feeling tired and cold. In the 'traditional medical interview' the doctor takes a careful history and examination and arranges investigations for such conditions as anaemia and myxoedema. The tests are normal, so a long interview of the 'detective inspector' type is arranged. The patient finds out quite a bit about the frustrations of her life and is grateful for this insight and the prescription of antidepressants, but returns worse rather than better. In the 'flash type interview' which followed, the patient burst into tears early on. The doctor's immediate reaction was that she

> *looked ridiculous crying while wearing a 'formidable'*
> *hat. He then realised that others might feel similarly*
> *unsympathetic towards this woman. The doctor suggested to*
> *the patient that she might be keeping people at arms' length*
> *and he felt able to refer to the hat. The patient accepted this*
> *feedback and offered the suggestion herself that her feelings*
> *of being cold might be because there was nobody to warm*
> *her up but that her stern manner was hiding this need from*
> *other people.*

Here the simple feedback offered by the doctor appears to have given rise to a whole new understanding - *felt* as well as *known* – by the patient. No doubt the interaction had the enormous bonus for the doctor that his understanding of the patient allowed him immediately to shed his feelings of frustration about her and maybe even to come to like her.

It is this sense of understanding which I firmly believe is what most patients want from their doctor (and, of course, the traditional medical model can be an essential part of the process). So often we (and I include myself here) are tempted to reassure instead of trying to understand. Needless to say, it is likely to be ourselves who are reassured, not the patient. In the same way when we, as doctors, have difficulty in our work with patients, we also want understanding rather than reassurance from colleagues:

Case history 8

At a case discussion group for GP registrars, deliberately run
without a leader, a case was presented of a woman with
vague symptoms of discomfort in her throat. The registrar
had been uncertain what to do and was also somewhat
angry that her trainer had more or less pushed her into

seeing this patient who was known to be difficult. In the end the doctor decided to refer the patient to an ENT surgeon, even though she had seen one previously and had had negative investigations. Group members spent a few minutes reassuring the presenter that there was little else she could have done and that they would have done the same thing. She did not seem convinced.

This discussion was in marked contrast to the one I mentioned earlier (case history 4), when the registrars had been led by an experienced course organiser. On that occasion the registrars also reassured the presenter that she had done nothing wrong, but the leader urged them to accept the presenter's anxiety and explore it. The 40-minute discussion opened up many areas of understanding about the doctor's relationship with the patient, his relatives, her training practice and, as mentioned earlier, her father.

It is this real understanding and support that is the gain from attending a well run case discussion group, or Balint group. Doctors (or other health professionals) participating in such a group are in many ways in an analogous position to patients attending the doctor. They want to explore and understand their feelings even if, at first sight, they may seem to be looking for quick reassurance or a prescription for action. Our wish for a quick solution is understandable, as some of the most critical aspects of our work, such as treating emergencies, *do* require rapid action. When dealing with feelings, however, this approach can be counterproductive and a group that spends too much time offering action plans is unlikely to be satisfying in the long term.

Every patient seen in general practice will give rise to some feelings in the doctor being consulted. If, on the one hand, these feelings are suppressed or left unresolved, they can give rise to stress in the doctor, which is likely to be made worse by an unsatisfactory outcome for the patient. If, on the other hand, the doctor's and patient's feelings are explored and understood, the outcome for both could well be transformed. Unfortunately the culture of the NHS at present makes it hard to put feelings to the top of the agenda. It is deeply disturbing that, for all the advantages of instant access, NHS Direct and Walk-in centres address patients' wants rather than their needs. To make things worse, doctors' attention is being focused on to such activities as health commissioning, rationing and screening. We can only hope that patients (i.e. all of us) will soon demand that the NHS does more to meet their real needs.

References

1 Balint M (1957) *The Doctor, His Patient and The Illness.* Pitman, London. 2e reprinted (1995). Churchill Livingstone, Edinburgh.

2 Salinsky J and Sackin P (2000) *What Are You Feeling, Doctor? Identifying and avoiding defensive patterns in the consultation.* Radcliffe Medical Press, Oxford.

3 Neighbour R (1987) *The Inner Consultation.* Kluwer Academic Publishers, Lancaster.

4 Balint E and Norell J (1973) *Six Minutes for the Patient.* Tavistock Publications, London.

Useful address

Dr David Watt, Secretary, Balint Society, Tollgate Health Centre, 220 Tollgate Road, London E6 4JS, UK.

Among other activities, the Balint Society holds one or two weekends per year at which doctors and other health professionals can have a taste of the type of case discussion group mentioned in this chapter.

7 Looking after yourself

Kevork Hopayian

Introduction

At first, I felt a hypocrite when I agreed to write this chapter. When I came to read it later, I was reassured to discover a list not only of my weaknesses but also of my strengths. So too, I imagine, will you: Poachers can make good gamekeepers.

Do not read this chapter passively. You should use it as a checklist to assess your present performance and as a guide to future action. It outlines a collection of measures which provide a comprehensive programme of emotional and mental hygiene. To get the most out of it, you must do more than just read it. Note the points that are relevant to you, come back to them, analyse the problems and plan your solutions.

The measures are classified under the headings: organisation, looking after yourself and relaxation.

Organisation

Managing time

Two items crop up whenever GPs grumble: too much work and too little time. I have been to a number of management training sessions where management consultants take this as proof of poor organisation and proceed to trot out a standard list of organisational principles. I will not repeat the calumny; you would not have got to be a GP if you were disorganised. But that does not mean that there is no room for improvement in the organisation of life for any of us. Organisation of life? Should that not be organisation of the practice? No!

To organise is to create a system that achieves your aims (to be effective) while using the least resources (to be efficient). Time is a precious resource, especially for a service like ours which is provided through people. So organisation means managing time, and that includes getting the right balance between work and home. Forgive me if *I* now trot out some organisational principles.

There are four steps in planning time:

1 choose your objectives
2 determine a plan
3 for each objective, draw up a timetable
4 review progress.

Most people rarely express their objectives in life formally, but there are times when it is immensely helpful. Here is an example, which demonstrates an attempt to balance personal and professional objectives.

- Family:
  - spend most evenings and weekends with family
  - support spouse in developing her career.
- Home:
  - improve garden.
- Surgery:
  - expansion of nurses' role
  - maintain income
  - contain inappropriate demands on practice.
- Education:
  - improve knowledge of rheumatology
  - pursue practice-based projects.
- Personal:
  - learn to swim properly.

- RCGP:
  - assist RCGP faculty to achieve plan
  - increase RCGP district activity.

Make a plan for each objective: detailing the projects, the resources needed and a deadline for each task. You will end up with a timetable and a list of tasks. Although much of the GP's work (e.g. surgeries) is fixed, and some of it is wholly unpredictable, there remains a lot of work that would benefit from being planned.

There is no one tool to manage time that suits everyone. It does not matter whether you use a pocket book, a diary, an electronic organiser or a palm-top computer, so long as you keep in sight your objectives, plans and timetable. The personal organiser and electronic organiser have the advantage of keeping everything (including addresses and phone numbers) together.

My preferred method is the personal organiser. I have divided my personal organiser into sections, for example, home, surgery, RCGP, where I keep notes and plans; I keep a separate section for tasks and their deadlines (a To Do list). I update the To Do list every few days, and use the diary section for appointments and as a reminder for deadlines.

To put all minor tasks on a To Do list would be tedious, especially if they are repetitive tasks, I usually keep a pile of them, such as letters to be dictated, to one side and deal with them at their allotted time or during a free moment, should it arise.

Is the effort spent on managing time worth it? Yes!

- Things get done.
- Less time is wasted.
- Jobs are kept in perspective and seem less daunting.
- You feel more in control of events.

This helps to maintain both a sense of perspective and a feeling of control, which stave off that feeling of being overwhelmed when demands are numerous and great.

Managing workload

External load

How much control do you have over the demands made on you? In group discussions, I have heard many GPs answer 'none' – we cannot control the demands made by patients, rising expectations or governments forcing perpetual change. This amounts to entrenched helplessness, dwelling on what is beyond our control to the point of ignoring what is not. There are many things we *can* control, such as list size, how we respond to patient demand, and whether or not we take on non-NHS work. Here is a real example.

After a housing association took over responsibility for council housing from our local district council, it sought to fend off disgruntled clients on the waiting list by recommending they get medical certificates. Within a few weeks we were bombarded with wholly inappropriate requests. We wrote to the association several times before we were able to reduce the demand. The time and effort expended was worth it, in the long term. It would have been easier, in the short term, to comply with these requests as some GPs did. Their motives were well intended but their actions misguided. Many of us confuse the natural desire to do the best for our patients with doing what we are asked. Saying no is hard and makes us feel guilty. However, the consequences of giving certificates on demand would be that they would lose their value, the patients with true medical grounds for rehousing would not get priority, and we would all be working harder to achieve nothing. Saying no was good for both our patients and ourselves.

Internal load

The internal organisation of your practice not only determines its effectiveness and efficiency but it also profoundly affects your personal workload and stress. Three principles are of particular relevance in stress: decision making, division of labour and delegation.

Decision making

Decision making refers to how a practice determines its objectives and plans. The principles of managing time also apply here, but there are two additional principles: you need to make clear who is involved in the decisions and who performs the tasks.

Division of labour

Involving partners and staff whenever appropriate makes it easier for the objectives to be understood and supported by all. The ensuing discussion allows problems to be explored fully, promotes the sharing of problems and can support individuals. A named person must be made responsible for specific tasks. Not every partner needs to be involved in every decision or task. Indeed, sometimes no partner need be involved, except in a supervisory role. Duplication and overinvolvement only sap energy, without promoting efficiency. Avoid this by dividing areas of responsibility and tasks between partners and staff.

Delegation

Delegate every task that does not need your expertise or presence. I remember one management training session where a GP pinpointed arranging hospital admissions in the middle of surgery as a major source of stress; at that particular hospital at that particular time, one could be holding the line for half an hour before reaching the house officer. She had not considered this possibility of delegating the task to a receptionist until others in the group pointed it out.

The value of such meetings lies in recognising that GPs already possess relevant skills and can build on their experience by learning from each other. Talking to other practices about common problems can be a fruitful way of sharing ideas and solutions, even when practices are so different. There are several models of practice organisation and the one that suits yours will depend upon size, personalities and commitments. The specifics of the model are not as important in the success of an organisation as much as how the basic principles are applied.

Looking after yourself

Social psychologists have demonstrated that emotional support, from a spouse, friends or colleagues, protects against stress. General practice can either destroy or provide supportive networks. There are many reasons for having a life outside work and for putting equal time and effort into fostering good relations with colleagues and friends, but one good reason is that not doing so leaves you isolated and vulnerable. Your behaviour towards others influences their behaviour towards you. There is a danger of a downward spiral when under stress: if you become irritable and repeatedly take out your anger on the nearest person, or if you become withdrawn and sullen, you risk estranging the very people whose support you need. Moreover, how others behave towards you can either undermine or reinforce your own sense of worth.

A sense of worth in what we do is important for how we feel about ourselves. This ties in with setting objectives. Set them unrealistically high and you commit yourself to exhaustion and disappointment. Set them too low and you sentence yourself to boredom and frustration. You may have met GPs who moan that general practice is boring because it is stuffed with trivia. They have set their sights so low that they confine themselves to the most facile work and miss the challenges that general practice poses. Their perception of practice diverges widely from that of GPs who enjoy and take pride in their work. Some GPs augment the value of their work by involvement in wider networks, such as RCGP groups, medico-political works such as Local Medical Committees, and young practitioner groups. This does not imply that they find practice boring. On the contrary, such GPs are enthusiastic about

general practice but their objectives extend beyond the daily round
of work. For example, medical politics brings a sense of control,
while educational groups fan the flames of enquiry.

The premise that our thoughts and perceptions influence our
emotions is basic to cognitive psychology. This hypothesis was
developed by clinical psychologists treating depression and anxiety,
but it is more widely relevant and well worth studying. Sufferers of
emotional disorder have similar distortions in their thinking and
perception (a list of the common types is shown in Table 7.1).
Therapists help patients to identify their distortions and to
replace them with more rational alternatives. Unlike psycho-
analysts, clinical psychologists do not claim that everyone needs
therapy. However, all of us at some time or another, particularly if
we are already feeling low, have negative images and beliefs about
ourselves as doctors which, left unchecked, can make us feel even
lower. Let me give a personal example. I once diagnosed pityriasis
versicolor in a new patient and in answer to direct questions, I
replied that the fungus is a commensal and transmission is from
person to person. She then saw a partner of mine to complain that I
had implied that she was promiscuous. I felt terrible and developed
irrational beliefs, of which the strongest was that I must be a useless
communicator. I went on to remember past misunderstandings
and felt worse. I got out of my negative thinking by identifying and
correcting my cognitive distortions:

1   overgeneralisation – even if I had communicated badly in this
    case, I was wrong to think that I do so in all cases
2   mental filter – I was only picking out the bad cases from the
    past, which, to be truthful, were exceptional
3   emotional reasoning – I felt useless and took this to be proof
    that I was.

Replacing my negative self-talk with positive self-talk stopped me
feeling terrible. Its purpose, though, is not to dismiss problems but
to put them in perspective. (When her former notes eventually
arrived, I discovered that this particular patient had a long record

Table 7.1 Common cognitive distortions (taken from Burns (1980)[1])

1 All-or-nothing thinking
   You see everything as all or nothing. Your performance has to be perfect; if you fail in one way, you see yourself as a total failure.

2 Overgeneralisation
   You see a single failure or bad event as proof of a repetitive pattern in your life.

3 Mental filter
   You pick out negative details and dwell on them so much that you cannot notice anything else.

4 Disqualifying the positive
   You can always find a reason to reject positive experiences. You end up ignoring all the positive things in your life.

5 Jumping to conclusions
   You draw negative conclusions even in the absence of proof. There are two ways of jumping to conclusions:
   (a) mind reading; you assume someone has a downer on you without checking facts
   (b) fortune telling; you anticipate that things will turn out badly and act as if your prediction is a fact.

6 Magnification or minimisation
   You exaggerate the importance of negative things, such as your weak points, and underestimate the importance of positive things, such as your strengths.

7 Emotional reasoning
   You assume that your emotions truly reflect the way things are, e.g. 'I feel useless so I must be'.

8 Should statements
   You try to motivate yourself with shoulds and should nots, resulting in guilt. When you direct should statements at others, the result is anger and frustration.

9 Labelling and mislabelling
   Labelling is an extreme type of overgeneralisation where you stick a negative label onto a person because of a negative event. You can label yourself, 'I'm useless' or others 'He's selfish'. Mislabelling goes one step further and uses emotionally charged labels.

10 Personalisation
   You see yourself as the cause of negative events even though you have little or no control over them.

of making false accusations against doctors.) Recognising and admitting that we make mistakes in communication and other aspects of our work (and recognising that we do so more commonly when the pace or duration of work is excessive) is useful and constructive; allowing ourselves to be overwhelmed by feelings of doubt and guilt is unhelpful and destructive.

Let me outline a nightmare of a day: read post, hold morning surgery, write repeat scripts during coffee break, home visits, lunchtime – no longer than it takes to eat a sandwich – factory session, hold evening surgery, write repeat scripts while having tea, dictate letters, go home still in fifth gear and engine overheated before starting on call or setting off to an evening meeting. Far-fetched? No, I have done days like that and no doubt so have you. It can be done; we adapt to the pace. Adapting to an increased load by working faster and for longer is a constructive response, so long as you do not let it become the norm. If you continue at too fast a pace for too long, your efficiency is bound to drop because there is no period for recovery. You enter the phase of decompensation: your efficiency drops, you find yourself falling behind and so push yourself even harder, only to become increasingly tired and inefficient. Which brings us back to time management. A timetable must include breaks for rest and recreation.

Avoid stimulants as an alternative to rest. Caffeine only post-pones exhaustion, it does not abolish it. While this may be valuable at times, caffeine has the same dangers as any stimulant drug: toxicity, tolerance and habituation. The toxic effects of caffeine (palpitations, anxiety, irritability and headaches) resemble some of the symptoms of stress and so may pass unrecognised. Caffeine has a long plasma half-life, so even if drunk during the day, plasma concentrations at night may be sufficient to disturb sleep, leading to further fatigue and a greater demand for caffeine. The culpable dose varies from person to person but starts as low as 500 mg a day, the equivalent of six cups of strong coffee. Coffee contains about 60–80 mg caffeine per cup, tea 20–40 mg per cup, and a can of cola about 25 mg. Take a break when you are tired or, better still, before you get tired and save your favourite drink for enjoyment. If there really is so much to do that you cannot have a break – stand back, take stock and investigate what has gone wrong.

Similarly, avoid using alcohol as a tranquilliser. If you regularly use alcohol to wind down after a day's work or to help you get to sleep – stand back, take stock and find out why you need to do so. If you need to wind down, consider alternatives such as relaxation techniques or physical exercise.

Long working hours and fatigue are reasons given by many of our patients for rejecting our advice to exercise more. It is so easy for us to fall into the same trap. There are several possible explanations for the benefit of exercise: physiological adaptation improves stamina, exercise is a diversion from work, or it may be simply the benefit of recreation. Whatever the reason, schedule some form of regular exercise into your timetable. You need to exercise frequently to maintain physical fitness. Avoid infrequent, long sessions because they are more likely to lead to injury than frequent, short sessions. Occasional squash players beware! It is easier for those who enjoy sport and do it as a hobby, but the rest of us can always find some activity to suit.

Relaxation

Spending time on a hobby or pastime can be relaxing, either by taking time out from work (diversion) or by enjoying oneself (recreation), but it is not always so. Juggling was extremely fashionable in the early nineties, especially among business people (yuppie yoga?) with claims for its unique properties. Its exit from fashion illustrates that it is not so much what you do as the value of diversion and recreation. However, some exercises aim specifically to induce profound states of relaxation. They have been part of life for various peoples for centuries and more recently have been used successfully to treat clinical anxiety.

They vary from the very simple, such as listening to music, through to skills such as self-hypnosis and finally to whole philosophies, such as imported Eastern religions. Each has its ardent supporters, but there is no evidence that any one is superior. They have a common core; focused attention and suspension of critical thought. These open the door for entry into an altered state of consciousness (ASC). In an ASC, left cerebral hemisphere activity diminishes and the right hemisphere becomes dominant, recognised on the electroencephalogram through prominent alpha-waves. What does an ASC feel like? Relaxing, refreshing, rapturous. We experience them spontaneously; relaxation exercises allow us to summon them when needed or wanted.

In hypnosis, a second person helps by giving suggestions. The same processes are used in yogic meditations (they include: concentration on a fixed point (Dharana), muscular relaxation (Savasana), alteration of perception (Pratyahara), breath control (Pranayama) and visualisation (Dhyana)), but here you are on your own. Doctors and clinical psychologists who practise hypno-therapy teach patients self-hypnosis in order to maintain their autonomy, in contrast to the many relaxation tapes on sale which consist of instructions spoken in a soothing voice to background music. Autogenic training was developed by clinical psychologists who disliked hypnosis; the steps are so similar to self-hypnosis that the difference is lost on me. Transcendental meditation is one form of yogic meditation which has been commercially packaged.

Ignore the hype, choose what suits you best. For starters, here are two relaxation techniques which are free and can be learnt from the written word.

Self-hypnosis

Lie or sit in a comfortable position. Shut your eyes and notice the comfort that it brings. Now concentrate on each part of your body in turn and tell yourself that you feel it relax. Start with your feet; feel them, be aware of them, let them fill your consciousness and tell yourself they are relaxing. Move up the body, calves, knees, thighs and so on, finishing with neck, scalp, temples and then the face. By then you may well have induced hypnosis. Deepen the hypnotic state by any or all of the following techniques:

- Count from 1 to 10, telling yourself that with each count you become one degree more relaxed.
- Focus on your breathing, feel your chest expand and deflate, and tell yourself that you are becoming more relaxed with each exhalation.
- Use visual imagination. One example is to imagine a white, cleansing mist that enters your body when you inhale and takes away any tension left in your body when you exhale.

If you find this too hard at first, make a tape-recording of the suggestions. This is preferable to buying a ready-made tape because, from the outset, your aim is to perform the exercise independently. When proficient you can perform it anytime, anywhere, anyplace.

Alternate nose breathing

This is a very simple but effective yogic exercise. Shut your eyes. Place one index finger, say your right index finger, on your forehead. Close the right nostril with your thumb. Inhale slowly through the left nostril while counting slowly to four. With your middle finger also close the left nostril and hold your breath to the count of four. Finally, release your thumb and exhale through the right nostril to the count of four. Complete the round by repeating the steps starting with the right nostril. Perform several rounds.

The next step

If you have read this far without finding any faults in yourself, read no more. In fact, you ought to revise this chapter for the next edition. If you have recognised some areas of improvement, start as you mean to go on: draw up your plan now!

Reference

1 Burns DD (1980) *Feeling Good.* Morrow and Company, New York.

Further reading

Hewitt J (1992) *Teach Yourself Yoga.* Hodder and Stoughton, London.

WHO (1980) *On Being in Charge. A Guide for Middle-level Management in Primary Health Care.* World Health Organization, Geneva, Switzerland.

8 How to cope with stress in one's partners, and in the practice

Tom Davies

Prevention is better than cure.

Introduction

The most important factor in dealing with the topic of stress is the simple acknowledgement that modern general practice is a very stressful job. The responsibilities, the constantly increasing demand (for 24 hours a day), with the ever-important need to keep up to date, both with the medical and technological developments, all take their toll. Many GPs liken modern practice to trying to keep going on an ever faster turning treadmill. Change continues apace. *No one is immune from stress.* Indeed, those GPs who deny that they are stressed may well be those who most need help. Incidents that can trigger feelings of anxiety or a major depression may be trivial in themselves. It is easy, within the practice, to laugh at some of these events (humour is, of course, a well-recognised way that people cope with stress), but for the partner concerned this might be the last straw. This is particularly true of complaints, which despite often having no substance at all, can still affect the partner significantly.

Box 8.1   General points to avoid stress

- Recognise that no one is immune.
- Acknowledge that general practice is a stressful job.
- Trigger events may be trivial, and not noticed by partners.
- Particularly need to take complaints (however trivial, unheralded) seriously and sympathetically.
- Don't take things personally.

Complaints

Complaints are a major contributory factor to stress in general practice and warrant a chapter by themselves (Chapter 12). Many GPs now feel that things have gone too far, and that the system is far too one-sided in favour of the patient, who is at liberty to make the most frivolous and unjustified complaint. The doctor is left, often for months, with the worry of wondering about the outcome, often still being responsible for the care of the complainant and his or her family. When the doctor is cleared there are never any apologies from the family, and morale inevitably falls. It is essential that all partners are aware when any complaints are made, both to support the affected member of staff, and also so that the situation isn't accidentally exacerbated. A suitable discrete record should be made in the medical record.

Prevention

The basis for any good relationship is that of trust and complete honesty. Partners need to feel valued. Great care should be taken to ensure an equal workload and sharing of the responsibilities. Work needs to be properly delegated. Undoubtedly there is nothing that, potentially, will cause greater unhappiness than an unequal work-load (or the feeling that work is not properly shared). There should be frequent, regular meetings; in our own practice that means two a week, in addition to the impromptu meetings, which all partners try and attend before and during surgeries (see later). One meeting is specifically educational, with partners taking it in turn to lead the meeting. These are interdisciplinary meetings with our nurses and health visitors. The other meeting every week is to discuss the business and administrative side of the practice. An agenda is produced, and simple minutes (action points) kept to ensure that there are no misunderstandings, and for absent partners to keep up with all the decisions being made. The chairman of the meeting may be changed regularly, again to ensure that everyone is seen to be playing an active part in the practice. A further refinement of this is to delegate an area of responsibility to each doctor, so that one partner takes responsibility for the treatment room, education and library, computers and technology or drugs and buildings – being examples used in our practice. These responsibilities may rotate after set periods of time.

Box 8.2 Prevention

- Build on trust, honesty.
- Remove causes of unhappiness; avoid feelings of unequal work/rewards.
- Must encourage delegation of duties.
- Relax positively. Family crucial (but often under-valued, and practice work may be resented).
- Community work/extracurricular work important, but needs to be rationed.
- The GP should register with another practice.
- Holidays are important. All partners should have equal rights and priority.

- Acknowledge a trade-off between rewards and peace of mind (extra work may bring in extra income, but at what price?).
- Consider regular (?annual) individual partner appraisals. Positive feedback.
- Protected time, to be able to concentrate in an uninterrupted way on one item (also true of family time).

Regular meetings may be seen as yet another intrusion on a busy day, but I do believe that they ensure that real opportunities exist to share ideas and, at times, to have frank discussions of potential problem areas. A fly on the wall at our practice meetings may be surprised at the strength of feelings sometimes expressed, but once out, they are dealt with and everyone can move forward. They certainly can't be dealt with if kept suppressed. GP registrars in the past have expressed surprise at the banter across the table, which at times gets quite heated. However, with different strong personalities involved, all with positive ideas, without such a mechanism the potential for unresolved issues to create resentment would be very real and problems would quickly arise. It is very easy for such meetings always to be negative, and positive suggestions should be the rule. Good chairmanship should ensure that views from all are heard. Where a presentation is made, the partner responsible must be given full time to make the presentation, and care taken to enhance the good points first (Pendleton's Rules).

Several partnerships have started to introduce individual partner appraisals, sometimes with partners pairing off. This is a technique used increasingly by management, which sounds threatening, but actually gives partners time to work together, and can have surprisingly positive pay-offs.

Box 8.3   Regular meetings

- Hold them frequently and regularly.
- Have an agenda. Keep to topics, stay to time. Don't dwell on trivial issues.
- Minute them (avoid misunderstanding).
- Appoint a chairman (consider rotating).
- Use Pendleton's Rules.
- Look at equal distribution (and responsibilities) for management areas in the practice.

Protected time

An important concept for modern general practice is that of protected time. Despite one's best intentions, it is difficult, when emergencies need to be dealt with, to avoid interruptions. In our practice we have attempted to have away days, and even on one occasion an away weekend, with the work being covered by a reliable locum. This was very successful, and much productive work took place, with us all feeling suitably refreshed and recharged with ideas. The down side of these arrangements tends to be the disruption of one's family time. Consequently, we have arranged to take a working afternoon within the practice once every three months, with the surgery only open for emergencies, covered by a locum. So far this seems to be the ideal solution. Increasingly these meetings involve all members of the primary care team, with opportunities to have open and frank discussions away from the pressures of emergencies and patients clamouring to be seen.

Time away from the practice

Everyone should have the opportunity to unwind, and pursue some activity outside medicine. This should be active and not just passive. Just getting home and switching off is not enough. Ideally, such pursuits can be carried out with members of the family. Sport, gardening, music, reading may all be used to recharge one's batteries. The question of work outside the practice is more difficult. This can be both stimulating and challenging for the doctor concerned, and many practices allow partners equal time away to pursue activities, which may be both local (industrial medicine, clinical assistants, committees such as the LMC, MAAG, RCGP faculty) and national. GPs must play their part in national committees, and represent the very poorly understood part of the profession. One's consultant colleagues, unless they have spent time in general practice, often don't have a clue. The voice of the GP should be heard, and if more work is to come to general practice, resources must then follow. Care must be taken to agree on an equitable distribution of money earned outside general medical services. A partner taking time off and earning extra money in 'practice time' from work done when others are working harder looking after patients could easily be the recipe for the build-up of much resentment.

Undoubtedly, the low morale in the profession at the present time is itself a major stress factor. However, the problem with all out-of-practice commitments is the time it takes the doctor away from his or her patients and the stress it puts on the partnership. The financial rewards will seldom justify the time away, with reimbursement covering either just travel, or a small amount to cover a locum. The partners may be left with the view that they are, in effect, subsidising the organisations involved, never mind how worthy. In an ideal world, all partners should be doing an identical amount of work, both in and away from the practice, but this is almost impossible. The issues that time out of the practice raise must be faced. At times partners will require one member of the group to cut back on the outside work, not to spite him, but to prevent that partner 'blowing a fuse'.

GPs are not good at saying no, and a partner may be grateful to have the ability to say no, because of the practice's agreement.

Social activities should also be considered for the practice. One often sees one's partners in a different light away from the 'coalface'. Inter-practice meetings, at sport or some form of quiz, can enable the feeling of pulling together. Undoubtedly one's staff enjoys the chance of seeing colleagues let their hair down and apparently being 'more human'.

The working day

In our practice we have constantly strived to identify the problem areas: the number of appointments available, how long they should be, how to deal with the telephone and other interruptions. Here good reception and administrative staff are invaluable, and can take an appreciable amount of work away from the doctors. The timetable can be flexible, with catch-up periods in-built, enabling the doctor to feel less stressed because of running late. The nurse, or dispensary, may well be able to deal with a lot of the queries that originally may have presented as a request for an appointment. In some practices with a high home visiting schedule, this may be purely the case because no surgery appointments are readily available in the short term. The telephone, although an intrusion, can be used very effectively to save time. Many practices increasingly agree to receive calls, or return them at set times. Nurse triage is gaining favour as an effective way of filtering demands. Talking directly to a patient or patient's relative is very much more satisfactory than leaving messages, or risking building up resentment in the patient when they 'couldn't get an appointment'. Patient pressure remains one of the most stressful aspects of the business of general practice, particularly for the reception staff.

Good communications within the practice are essential. Admissions, deaths and serious diagnoses all need to be shared with one's partners (where possible, if the hospitals play their part) so that one is forewarned for dealing with relatives, friends, etc.

Doctors are notorious for ignoring their own health needs, and every GP should be registered with a GP away from the practice. This can be difficult in very isolated areas, but colleagues inevitably are sensitive to the problem and will take doctors and their families onto their list from 'outside their practice area'. Junior partners may feel threatened on joining a practice where it has been the norm for the families to register with their own practice, but should, where possible, resist the pressure to register.

The single partner may, on entering general practice, feel increasingly isolated from his or her peers who have remained in hospital medicine, or moved away. Young practitioners' groups are excellent methods of dealing with problems that face all young doctors. Doctors may be under pressure at certain times, particularly at times of change. Key times include when there may have been a birth or death in the family. Moving house is a well-recognised stressful event, as is of course divorce, which may be the effect of stress as well as the cause of more stress. Partners (and other members of staff) are well advised to try to keep an open eye on these matters, to minimise the potential for conflict. Often, partners will not want to admit any problems, but will be grateful for the opportunity to share such problems if asked. The practice may not be the ideal stage for such a discussion, and time may need to be set aside to meet out of hours, maybe in a local pub.

Box 8.4 Identify higher risk person

- Socially isolated.
- Recent bereavement/loss.
- Perfectionist personality.

The practice contract

A good practice contract is essential. It still happens that many practices do not have a practice contract ('We don't need such a thing here, we all trust one another') and it is not a helpful or realistic attitude. The practice and partners need to be very clear about the arrangements for sickness cover. Who pays for the locums? When are they brought in? How long may a partner be off work? What happens when he or she returns and is subsequently ill? If the partners have to do extra nights, are they recompensed on a 'locum' basis? After a lengthy time off, a partner may well wish to come back on a part-time basis. The practice should be supportive of such an arrangement, but once the partner is working even for the briefest time, the sickness cover covering their absence will stop, and hence the practice may be financially worse off. It is possible to come to an arrangement by using part of one's holiday entitlement to come back on a flexible part-time basis. The use of local occupational health services (if available) is also helpful, although unfortunately not always accepted by the sick colleague. Confidentiality with using such services is still perceived as a potential problem, especially with the high levels of psychosocial problems and substance abuse that occurs.

Box 8.5 Practice contract

- A practice contract is essential.
- It must stipulate sickness arrangements.
- There should be no financial loss (nor inducement!) to be off work.
- Consider whether the locum insurance/sickness premiums should be paid by the practice (a gesture of goodwill – low-premium junior partners will become high-premium older partners! Also tax deductable if a requirement of the practice contract).
- Holidays equal for all.
- Consider building in sabbatical arrangements for 'refreshment'.
- Honour study leave.

- Social activities.
- What notice will be required for permanent retirement?
- What about future illness. What is the formula for further time off following more illness?

The partner who is showing signs of stress

How does one become aware that there is a problem, or a potential problem, with a partner? A change in behaviour would be a key thing to note. This can be both a withdrawal, from meetings, from activities, avoidance of visits, seeing the urgent extra appointments, or a move to the other extreme where the partner takes on more and more, trying to prove that they are 'coping'. The receptionists and practice manager may have a greater opportunity to see the effects of the partner's behaviour on the surgery arrangements. The partner's timekeeping may become worse, there may be long gaps in between the patients being called. The attitude of the partner to other staff may change, with short-tempered responses. The patients themselves can also be very perceptive to such behaviour, requesting to see another doctor, and can, at times, be very frank and honest. Such views may be expressed to other partners. When presented with such information it is very easy to rationalise along the lines of 'so and so is having a bad day, he had a bad night', etc. This of course may be the case, but it may also be the first opportunity to recognise a problem, and a prompt for one of the partners to say something. Doctors are notorious in not recognising signs in colleagues that they might far more readily recognise in patients with regard to alcohol abuse or even drug dependence.

The partners may offer to take some of the work away from the stressed partner, but this is of course difficult, as it may reinforce feelings of inadequacy in the sufferer. The most important aspect of

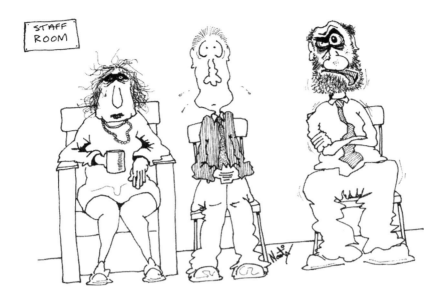

this situation is for there to be an admission that there is a problem. Until that happens the partners may themselves become increasingly stressed with what seems to be an impasse. It may be possible, ideally at a meeting away from the practice, for the partners to have a general discussion on stress, or pressures in the practice, giving examples from their own lives to try and draw the partner to discuss his or her feelings. It may well be that the cause of the stress may be an intolerable workload that can only be dealt with by taking in an extra partner, increasing hours of appointments, or changing the timing arrangements, so that there is more flexibility to deal with the time pressures. Outside commitments of all the partners need to be looked at regularly.

The partner may wish to cut back, and may request dropping to a part-time arrangement, at least in the short term. This may well be ideal, but other partners themselves may wish for something similar and it would be difficult to conceive of a practice which could accommodate all the partners in such an arrangement. Financial recompense will need to be made if the partner cuts back. To ask the others to do more, while the partner who is cutting back draws the same or even more (if seniority or other earnings are kept separately), would be invidious. Locums may be used in the short term to cover the work, but they are increasingly difficult to find, do not provide good continuity of care, and may well have difficulties with the increasingly complicated business of general practice, computers, etc.

Decisions need to be made about informing the staff of any changes, and why they are being implemented. Involving them in trying to pinpoint problem areas can be very important, both to make them feel valued but also to find real practical solutions. They may need to be told that Dr Bloggs is cutting back for a period and they should know how to handle such information confidentially. A sabbatical may be the way for all parties to refresh, but again cover will need to be provided, and financial reparation made.

Box 8.6   The partner who is still at work

- Does he or she recognise that there is a problem?
- Can his or her workload be reduced?
- How are the other partners affected?
- Clarify financial arrangements allowing the partner to put in a locum at their expense.
- Look at time-management skills.
- Look at distribution of work (clinical and administration should be fairly shared).

The partner who is away

This is the situation that most practices may wish to avoid, but if it does come about, it must be taken as an opportunity for the whole practice to take stock of what they are doing, and where they are. It may well be an ideal opportunity to examine some of the factors that may have contributed to the one partner's absence. Workload, appointments, etc. can all be looked at.

It is vital that contingency plans for illness exist, ideally drawn up well before anyone is away, so that decisions made are free from any danger of their being interpreted personally. There is no denying that illness, almost always occurring suddenly, is a major stressful event for the practice. The practice should be keen to stay in close touch with the absent partner, but endless visits by everyone concerned could be almost as unhelpful as a complete absence of visits. In this respect the remaining partners may see themselves in a 'no win' situation. Visits may be viewed suspiciously, 'Why are they coming round to check?', or if the partners choose to give the absent doctor some space, the comment may be made that the practice is uncaring and uninterested. How sensible it would be if the partners, before they ever become ill, were to say what they would wish regarding visits. It is very helpful, if possible, to have as open a dialogue as possible with the spouse, to try to discover what the partner might want.

Decisions must made with regard to what patients are told. In most instances something near the truth would be best, because ideally the partner should be out and about, and a story of a physical ailment may be viewed with some scepticism by patients. The practice grapevine should not be underestimated in such instances! The staff also need to be kept fully in the picture, both for their own piece of mind, but also to be able to brief patients.

Box 8.7   The partner who has time off

- Anticipate and make contingency plans.
- Discussions are much easier when they aren't personalised.
- What visiting/contact arrangements wanted? (Practice in a no-win situation. Support or harassment!)

- Involve spouse. Spouse may be particularly suspicious of motives.
- How can the practice enable a return to work (holiday compromise).
- Is it beneficial to be kept abreast of what is happening.
- What should one tell the staff and patients?

Inevitably, such an occurrence produces significantly extra work for the partners. The burden of out-of-hours calls, always one of the more stressful aspects of practice, will increase for the existing partners. In our practice, we now pay a nominal amount for the extra night cover, as indeed we also do to our part-time partners for extra surgeries that they cover. Obviously, the extra work should even itself out across all the partners, but in the short term, it is very stressful if one or two partners, stepping in at short notice, often to the detriment of the family, feel they are doing more than their fair share. It is but a small token, but can be very helpful. GP co-operatives taking over some of the out-of-hours duties may help in this respect, but financial arrangements for who pays when a partner is off must be clear. It is not recommended that partners should swap their on-call with colleagues while they are off sick, only to pay them back when they return to work.

Box 8.8   How to help the practice – strategies to cope

- Anticipate.
- Make locum payments to partners doing the work.
- Plan return to work. Use holiday entitlement to come back part-time.

- Practice (and absent partner) must keep in contact.
- Take out short-term insurance (practice/partner expense).
- All partners must have personal long-term insurance and pension arrangements.
- SS payments – don't forget to claim.
- Contact the health authority. Make a case for the need for locum employment (and reimbursement).

Conclusion

An increasing number of doctors are undoubtedly experiencing quite serious effects of stress. Some doctors have felt so desperate that they have committed suicide. It may be that, by nature, the type of person who chooses to become a GP is more vulnerable. To try to deal with all one's patients' troubles can become too much. Family and patients can suffer, and the vital support that might help may not be given, or wanted. It is absolutely right that every one of us should examine closely our own lifestyles and look around us at our colleagues to see if there are other things we should be doing.

9 Stress and the non-principal

Tina Ambury

What stress? You have no practice management hassles. You can choose when and how you work. You waltz in, see patients and leave at the end of surgery. Surely that's why you became a non-principal – to avoid stress?

So said a principal colleague of mine, succumbing to a common misconception, when he heard I was contributing to this book. And I had to agree with him – up to a point.

After all, when I stopped work for the birth of my daughter, I had serious doubts as to whether I would return to general practice, or medicine, at all. I had been a single-handed GP in the armed forces, working in a two-doctor practice. The stresses this placed on me, led to a threatened miscarriage. My staff and family also felt the strain. The fact that I looked forward to motherhood as a chance for a rest, only goes to show how bad things had got.

Of course, when the time came, I realised I wasn't cut out to be an earth mother – it was just as stressful! – and I decided to go back to work. The only certainties were that I did not want to work full-time and that out-of-hours work was out of the question.

My options were also limited by my husband's job requiring us to move house on an almost yearly basis. My only prospects were as a non-principal. But why should non-principals be any different to other GPs when it comes to stress?

It is certainly true that non-principals work flexibly; I plan my sessions around my family and other commitments. It is also true that I can walk away from the work at the end of a session and am not involved in the day-to-day business management of any of the practices I work in. But to say the life of a non-principal is stress-free is simply not true. We merely have different stressors. Some of these are obvious, others less so.

Money, money, money

Job and financial insecurity are facts of life for non-principals, sometimes painful and worrying ones. It is all well and good limiting the number of sessions you want to do in a week to stay flexible, but what happens when the phone doesn't ring?

Women's problems

As most non-principals are working mums, all the stressors alluded to in Kate Wishart's chapter on women about stereotyping at work and the home–work interface also apply.

You are not alone – you just think you are

Non-principals, especially those not attached to a particular practice, are isolated both professionally and educationally. In addition to the stress isolation itself can cause, in these days of impending revalidation non-principals often feel excluded from the processes of continuing professional development and fear this will prevent them from meeting the requirements of revalidation. This would ultimately mean losing their job and their livelihood.

Clinical and practice issues

Less obvious factors happen in the surgery itself. For non-principals, every patient is a new patient and may well take a considerable amount of time. Heartsink patients are notorious for doctor hopping and often seek out the locum – we are all aware how consultations with such patients can drag on.

Sometimes practices don't make things any easier, by dropping the non-principal in at the deep end, with no guidance on where things are, how the computer system works or what the referral pattern of the practice is. Non-principals find themselves wasting precious time searching for this information.

All this can lead to surgeries overrunning, with practices understandably unhappy about paying over the odds for a 'slow worker'. Deciding on the appropriate payment for work done always seems to generate stress – and women are not, in general, very assertive.

Strategy is the key – almost everything has been tried at least once before

As with all stress, there are ways of coping with, and even reducing, it. So where do you start? Unsurprisingly, the best way to reduce your stress levels is by forward planning – in the case of non-principals, this means even before you start looking for work.

Most non-principals know in advance when things will change, whether that be at the completion of vocational training or at the end of a period as a principal. Use this time well and the transition will go much more smoothly. Start by asking yourself the following key questions.

- *Where* do you plan to work?
- What do you *need* to earn?
- What do you *want* to earn?
- *What hours* would you like to do?
- Do you want to do *out-of-hours* work?

Know where you're at and where you want to be

You may think the 'where' may not be within your control, but think again. Do you want to work in rural or urban practices? Big or small? Computerised or not? The possibilities are endless, even if the geographical area tends to predominate in a particular kind of practice. What you should decide very early on, is how far you are prepared to travel to work. Quite apart from the issue of mileage-to-practice-boundary payments, do you really want to travel an hour before arriving? Worse still, could you cope with that extra hour before arriving home at the end of the day? If you have children to take care of (and most non-principals do), the cost of those early and late hours on the child-minding bill may negate any monetary benefit you would make by working so far away from home.

Children sweeten labours, but make misfortune bitter

Now might be a good point to talk about child-care. If non-principals are flexible, it is usually borne out of necessity – children can be both flexible and regimented. The only way a non-principal with parental responsibility can even consider working, is to ensure she (or he) has access to top-quality and above all, flexible, child-care. In the past I've been tied into the child-care trap of paying for a full-time place, even when I didn't use it, in order to retain the place. The situation is fraught with potential stressors and varies from one area to another. The best advice is simply to shop around before entering into any contract. The ideal of a carer who only charges for the hours they have your child, who will accept extra hours at the drop of a hat and who doesn't mind the frantic call saying surgery is running late, *is* out there – look well and negotiate.

Loads of dosh?!

The child-care issue will also obviously impact on how much you need to earn. There is no point slogging away full-time when most of the income goes in tax and child-care.

In reality, what you actually earn is a combination of three things: what you need, what would you like and what work is available.

The amount of work available, although dependent on what part of the country you work in, seems to be unlimited – especially in these days of increasing out-of-practice commitments. Having said that, it can be very hard to say no to a day's work in the hope that you might get a booking for a longer period later.

I found this so difficult when I first started non-principal work that I was soon working almost full-time. This meant less time for my family and struggling to complete my non-clinical work in the evenings. Although I've learnt to say no more often, I still worry that I won't find enough work when I move to a new area. Any combination of sessions is possible, including out-of-hours work. With a young family, I choose to work part-time, during 'office hours' only.

Once you have decided on your basic plan, you can then refine it. Because of my need for flexible daytime hours and my enforced mobility, I work freelance as a peripatetic locum. If you are more concerned about staying 'current' in practice, and have a defined period to work with, a retainer post or other practice-based assistant position might be more appropriate. Of course, you may choose that a high-earning out-of-hours job is for you. Whatever you decide, your next task is to sell yourself.

Communicate to accumulate

GPs or their practice managers can only offer you work if they know you exist and can contact you. Get yourself known. Put your name on the area's locum list – be that with the health authority, the PCG or local postgraduate centre. Phone or fax your details to local practices, as direct contact is often the best way of generating work and word of mouth on the practice manager network is very effective. Sitting back and waiting for the bookings to come in is naïve and inadvisable.

But once they do, a highly organised system is required. Practice managers often work through a list of preferred doctors when they require a locum. If time is tight and you are not home, they could very well move on to the next name. There is nothing more frustrating than getting home to a list of messages and, on returning the calls, discovering that they have found someone else to do the work. Having a mobile phone means they can contact you instantly, with the disadvantage of its possibly going off during a consultation. I find the combination of an answer-phone, a pager and a mobile phone (the number for which I don't give out) works well. My answer-phone message advises urgent callers to page me and, if they do, I can call them back between patients.

You must also beware the possibility of double booking. Once you confirm a booking, it is bad form to cancel except in emergency circumstances (which goes for the practice too). A work diary is essential. If you are as hopeless with paper as I am, investing in an electronic organiser is a sound investment. Mine has the capability of synchronising with my home PC to avoid a mismatch between the two.

Before confirming a booking, it is advisable to be certain what is being asked. Negotiating skills are a boon – don't price yourself out of work, but, at the same time, avoid selling yourself short. If possible, determine when you are needed, exactly what is expected of you and how much you will be paid for it, before ending the call. It is good business sense to follow up this conversation in writing as soon as possible.

Of course, even the best-laid plans fail at times and contingency plans are required for the unpredictable – like a child being unwell. Your working partner may need to shoulder some of the responsibility here, which may be made easier if current plans by the government to allow parents of children under five to take time off work are implemented fully.[1] However, I've found that most practices are remarkably understanding when the worst does happen, especially if you have a reputation for otherwise being reliable.

Education, personal development and support

So far, pre-empting business stress with good organisation has been my theme. Yet non-principals, like any GPs, will encounter their share of consultation-based stress, from worries about misdiagnosis to, plain and simply, difficult patients. Isolation rears its ugly head again here. It is often not possible to discuss cases with the team you are working for, and you may fear that your clinical skills are not as up to date as you would like. Remember, two (or more) heads are better than one. Attend postgraduate meetings in your area (this can also lead to work bookings) and join your local non-principal support group. Don't worry if there isn't one in your area, start one yourself – contact the National Association of Non Principals (NANP)[2] for information about this. Joining such a group is vital for keeping up to date. Not only do local groups often organise their own educational sessions, they are usually pretty au fait with what is happening on the local postgraduate scene. Just having someone in a similar position that you can call on to avoid the pitfalls of non-principal life, is a great stress buster.

The stress engendered by the uncertainty surrounding what form the revalidation process will take, is bound to effect *all* doctors – non-principals are not exempt from revalidation. The General Medical Council (GMC) is working hard to ensure that this process will not disadvantage any particular group of doctors, and intends to pilot its procedures before fully implementing them. But what can you do in the meantime?

Continuing professional development has always been a problem for non-principals, especially those without a practice base. Although trying to second-guess the final GMC process is itself stressful and would be foolhardy, you *can* take action now. Once again, forward planning is useful, from a whole-life or career point of view, rather than just the relative short-termism of revalidation. The best way to achieve this is by 'reflective practice'.

There is nothing new about reflecting on one's practice, and to some extent we all do it. We all have patients and situations that make us stop and think 'Am I happy that I know all I need to in this situation?', or 'How could that have gone better?'. Forward planning for revalidation involves writing these thoughts down and doing something about them – euphemistically called identifying and addressing your learning needs. This should personalise the content of a doctor's educational programme – a personal learning portfolio. Every UK non-principal can get such a portfolio from the NANP. In this way, reflective practice and needs-directed learning are perfectly suited to non-principals, whose working schedule may make other, more formalised, educational activities difficult.

The final blueprint for the revalidation process may be very different from that envisaged now, but by keeping such a portfolio, you are, at the very least, likely to be gathering a great deal of the required data, *now*, on a continuing basis, rather than worrying about what *might* be.

Why bother?

If general practice is so stressful, why do GPs continue to do it? The answer to this question is different for all GPs. It must be acknowledged that by opting out of the independent contractor–principal system of general practice, non-principals have recognised the stresses of that system and have taken an active choice in dealing with, or avoiding that stress.

That said, it is obvious from this chapter that being a non-principal is *not* an easy, stress-free option – it simply involves swapping one set of stressors for another, different set. However, the whole object of stress management is to be in control of your own destiny and, although total control is impossible, the flexibility of non-principal work gives you more than just the illusion of control. Remember:

- plan ahead:
  - hours
  - earnings
  - child-care
  - always have a contingency plan
- network and lessen isolation:
  - work contacts
  - use a top-quality communication system
  - education opportunities
  - peer group support
- make time for the things you enjoy:
  - family and friends
  - non-medical interests.

Above all, if despite all your forward planning you find the stress becoming too much of a burden so that you no longer enjoy general practice, rethink your life-plan and career. After all, in choosing to become a non-principal you have already made such a decision at least once before. The next time won't be so fraught with anxiety.

References

1 Department of Trade and Industry (1998) *Fairness At Work White Paper*, Chapter 5, Family Friendly Policies. The Stationery Office, London. http://www.dti.gov.uk/ir/fairness/part5.htm

2 National Association of Non Principals, Freepost (SCE5375), PO Box 188, Chichester, West Sussex PO19 1FP, UK. http://www.nanp.org.uk/

10 Stress and the seven ages of the GP

George Smerdon

Throughout a GP's career there is an expectation of stress. Until relatively recently, that expectation was focused at the start, with A levels, finals and vocational training probably being lumped together as the appropriate rite of passage. It was thought that successful completion of this training would set a young doctor up with a job for life, enormous job satisfaction and decent pay. The hoops and hurdles of the right job or scheme and postgraduate qualifications served to keep us up to the mark, with just enough pressure to assure the public that the medical profession was a rigorous, well-audited one. Little did the unsuspecting public realise what their doctors were going through to maintain this service in the face of quite extraordinary changes in general practice. The latest of the stream of white papers, *The New NHS: modern, dependable*, while aspiring to be the ultimate change for the better, presents yet another challenge. How can we meet this and manage the change?

The reality for most of us is that we are 'snorkelling' – submerged under the waterline of pressures of work, personal crises and professional concerns, with the snorkel tube representing our professional integrity (our lifeline) constantly under threat of being swamped by these pressures. The view through the mask represents the vision of what we are trying to achieve.

Most of the time we are okay, but it is that unforeseen, unplanned-for stress that sabotages our efforts. At all stages throughout our career as GPs, our lives have become increasingly complex and we have found ourselves in increasingly bad shape to deal with unforeseen stress. This does not have to be a sledge-hammer blow. Indeed, it can often be a relatively minor pressure, but it is the fact that it is unforeseen, unplanned for and somehow beyond our control that is crucial. It would be wrong to paint an entirely desperate picture, because by and large GPs are a resilient breed, built to take the strain and actually thrive on the rough and tumble of it all.

So what is going wrong?

I believe that it is the contemporary threat to our professional integrity and professionalism, with its consequent personal chaos, that is at the root of so many of our problems. Does any doctor really expect this when he or she enters practice? Many people have many different ideas about what is going on and how to cope with it, and I do not want to add to this confusion, but simply to offer a model that can be applied at any stage in a GP's career to try and help plan for those bad times. In *As you like it*, Shakespeare describes the seven ages of man, and I would like to propose a similar model for the seven ages of a GP.

- **Age 1**: 'At first the infant mewling and puking in the nurse's arms' – registrar.
- **Age 2**: 'Whining schoolboy with his satchel' – first year in practice.
- **Age 3**: 'The lover sighing like a furnace' – young principal, aged 30–40.
- **Age 4**: 'Soldier – full of strange oaths' – mature GP in his or her prime, aged 40–50.
- **Age 5**: 'Justice – in fair round belly' – handing on to the next generation, aged 50–60.
- **Age 6**: 'The sixth age shifts into the lean and slippered pantaloon' – retirement part one.
- **Age 7**: 'Last scene of all that ends this strange and eventful history' – retirement part two.

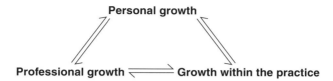

Figure 10.1   Model used for doctor appraisals.

What expectations of the problems of each age should we have? Each has pressures, some of which we should be, and indeed are, prepared for and actually embrace as being right, whereas others have less obvious problem areas which, if we could identify more clearly, we could go some way towards anticipating and developing a strategy or game plan which, even if it did not completely prepare us, might mitigate against some of the disasters that befall us, both professionally and personally.

In the doctor appraisals in our practice, we have found it helpful to use the model shown in Figure 10.1 when looking at not only what has happened in the previous year, but also what is expected in the future. I would like to demonstrate its use with regard to some of the seven ages of the GP's career.

Clearly, each doctor will need to apply their own concerns at whatever stage they have been through, or are going through, or are indeed approaching, but I believe that it is a simple, easy to apply and effective model. By considering the different ages of general practice, I would like to offer some examples to clarify use of the model. This is by no means intended to be a comprehensive examination of the issue, but more of an overview encouraging colleagues to give it a try.

Age 1: the registrar

So much depends on what sort of shape GP registrars are in and what their stress expectation is. Bad experiences in the hospital do have a profound influence on the rest of one's career as a GP, but most registrars are only too relieved to have reached their registrar year and are eager to get on with the job, little realising how much of the job has to be unlearnt and re-learnt.

Often they have been used to taking much responsibility in hospital jobs and now find it puzzling that it is difficult to take that responsibility, for all sorts of complex reasons (unplanned-for stress). At a personal level, registrars are still often of no fixed abode, but it is to their credit that they do not seem to mind this (expected or planned-for stress). Personal relationships with commitment have often been made by now and, again, any turbulence here has, to some extent, a built-in expectation of stress.

Where is the potential for development in the practice for registrars? The practice is not theirs and runs smoothly whether they are there or not! The uncertainty about how they fit in, in terms of a service commitment and how the practice is developing, can be very stressful for registrars, bringing with it the age-old tension of how nice to have an extra pair of hands and yet we must not exploit child labour (unplanned-for stress).

The emphasis here is on professional development. The registrars rightly expect and respond well to appropriate nourishment from their trainers, the practices in which they are working and their course organisers. What a registrar does not expect is to become disenchanted with general practice. All those years of commitment to a career and yet the reality does not match up to the expectation (sledgehammer blow). Neither do they expect to be abused, and there is no doubt that registrar abuse is something we all collude in, whether it is supporting unsatisfactory hospital jobs on a scheme, or things that go on in our practices that *we* know about, but which *they* are not expecting and therefore cannot plan for or cope with effectively. Often this abuse only surfaces later in professional life, but the wounds that have been inflicted and the damage that has been done can lead to considerable suffering.

The lifeline for the registrar is the expectation of finding the 'right practice'. It is to the credit of the training process that registrars no longer expect to find the 'perfect practice'. Stress expectation is high and many registrars prepare themselves for disappointment and failure. Applications are planned with meticulous care, with registrars even going on courses to make sure that they present themselves well. How then do registrars cope when they find that no practice wants them.

For a very small number, failing summative assessment will be a reality, and we are told that increasing numbers of registrars will probably not make it past this stage (sledgehammer blow).

There is no doubt that the process of summative assessment distorts the registrar year, creating tensions around submitting the video component and the audit project. Rationalising this and the MRCGP module into an extended 18-month attachment would ease many of these tensions. The learning potential seems increasingly marginalised by these pressures of the registrar. There is just so much to learn. Support and counsel for those who fail, and those for whom this pressure is a negative experience, needs to be more carefully thought about and appropriate mechanisms put in place.

Are some of the reasons why young doctors at the end of their training choose to become non-principals linked to the stress of the registrar year? It should be remembered that they also see how it is for partners in the practice with whom they are working. That sense of needing to be in control, or at least in contact with the helm, is a powerful force for most GPs, and the conscious decision to opt for the life of a non-principal is being made increasingly. However, for the purposes of this chapter, I see the majority of registrars going into partnership.

Age 2: young principal in the first year of practice

At this stage, development within the practice and personal development are predominant, but what is the stress expectation in these areas? Once in practice, the young principal is excited and keen to do well, wants to be liked by patients and colleagues –

create the right impression, yet retain the attractions of being the lad or lass.

Up until now I have avoided highlighting the different stresses that men and women experience, but it is probably important at this stage to state the obvious, that men and women do have different stress expectations, dependent on how they see their own personal development, their development within their chosen profession and their development within the new practice. This is dealt with in more detail in Kate Wishart's chapter. The practice looks to this new blood to revitalise things, bringing in new ideas with the energy of youth. The young principal expects life to change with the reality of full lists and shorter consulting times, combined with moving house and settling into a new area, with all the emphasis on personal development that this brings. Do we really adequately prepare the young principal for the stress expectation in these different areas? There is the muddle of the period of mutual assessment before the final decision is made – Should I stay? Shall we have him or her long term? Can we get the agreement sorted out? Is it worth the paper that it is written on? Who does the young principal turn to for guidance on this? They often find themselves unexpectedly alone. Spouses are often not in a position to understand the difficulties being experienced, as they are often in their own state of turmoil for sometimes similar, but often different, reasons. It really is a leap in the dark, with only good faith on the part of all concerned as the safety net, but is the good faith really there?

The youthfulness and energy is so often sabotaged by the practice and other partners:

- 'Yes – great idea, but we have tried it before and it didn't work, but do try it again if you want.'
- 'Of course, I was never a registrar, served my apprenticeship the hard way and there is nothing wrong with being thrown in at the deep end.' (Yes, there are GPs still saying this.)
- 'While you are about it, we are struggling a bit with the practice

formulary and updating our practice protocols; could you manage to sort these out?'
- 'We have been having a lot of trouble with our computer system and we thought that you were the whizz-kid that we were looking for.'

We could all find numerous examples of these put-downs that the young principals just don't expect and cannot plan for. However, it is likely that within the interactive model the young GP will be finding some nourishment for development and will probably have become quite adept at using the energy from the stronger development areas to offset the unexpected stresses that are being experienced. I hope that by now you are beginning to see how the model works.

Clinical governance formalises this development model, linking it not only to professional self-regulation and personal and practice development plans, but also to poor performance. The most common cause of this remains stress.

One of the partners in my trainee practice, simplistically I thought at the time, urged me to consider my future career and divide it into three decades. The first 10 years, roughly between the ages of 30 and 40, learning one's craft, then the next 10, between 40 and 50, firing on all cylinders – a regular Renaissance man – before entering the final decade towards retirement, passing the wisdom of one's experiences on to the young generation. In the final decade of my career I begin to understand what he meant.

Ages 3–5: doctors in general practice

As we embark on the third, fourth and fifth ages of general practice, what are the expectations of stress? What are we prepared for? What confronts us that we haven't planned for? As young principals we begin to learn what it is like to be pulled in lots of different directions. Our patients need us, our families need us, our practices need us and our careers begin to take on some shape. The conflicts may be unpredictable as we seek to find our way, looking to broaden our horizons with new professional interests. For young doctors, both men and women, with children, there is the tension between, on the one hand, wanting to be at home, especially in the early evening to be around to help when children are being put to bed, letting slip the events of their day; and, on the other hand, finding that evening surgery drags on with loads of urgent extra appointments, or finding that we have arranged a long 'last appointment' with a troubled patient needing more time.

What of women doctors? For many, the expectation of having children and all the pressure that this brings creates unexpected conflicts. Has an agreement been reached on maternity leave? Clearly, from the amount that is written about this, many women still find themselves up against it; along with the conflicts of doing what they feel ready to do and yet at the same time keeping their professional careers alive and honouring their commitment to their patients and to the practice.

It is easy to see how isolated a woman can feel, and many admit to feelings of guilt, sometimes generated from within themselves, but often generated by practice partners and even patients. Professional development and development within the practice often becomes suspended for them, but it does not seem to stop women doctors from developing very happy and effective careers as the years go by. Do women doctors burn out? The literature on stress in general practice is, of course, heavily weighted towards the male experience, but a major part of the expectation of stress for women GPs is how they learn to live with the men in their lives. As the number of women GP principals increases, it will be interesting to see what happens to the expectation of stress in this area of practice life.

Rather than separate off the pressures and problems of three decades of mature practice, I would like to introduce a longitudinal component to the interactive model, which reflects personal, professional and practice changes that we will have to address over the length of our careers. PCGs will, however, set annual programmes to look at this development and, depending on how well everyone works together, there should be less stress generated. Well-planned changes will always create pressure but, again, it's the expected/unexpected tension that changes pressure into damaging stress. This is not the place to expand on the comprehensive list of pressures, but to simply flag up some things that we might be prepared for.

All of us have our own crunch zones but, again, being confronted by them can be quite unexpected and painful. How do we sustain our enthusiasm? How do we cope with the ever-increasing problem of patient complaints, possible litigation, the strain of out-of-hours work and concerns for personal safety? The problem of increasing violence against doctors is something many doctors never expected to have to face. Of course, there is much to compensate for this, with the undoubted satisfaction that many aspects of our job brings. Areas of our work begin to interest us more and more. We need to stretch ourselves intellectually, to look imaginatively and innovatively at how we provide care for our practice populations as well as individual patients. The expectation of having to develop and maintain strong management skills and a sound business sense is at last being addressed. We are, however, not always prepared for the tensions that this can create, both at a personal and professional level. For some, there will be the desire to be involved politically with the provision of healthcare, and thank goodness someone is prepared to do that. With revalidation will come additional pressures, but it is to be hoped that the profession will see this as an important part of our professional development, hopefully managed supportively by the powers that be.

The expectation of stress as we set out to achieve all this is readily acknowledged. Disenchantment with the job is increasingly a reality and is leading significant numbers of GPs not only to seek to change their practices, but also to look outside general practice for new careers. We try to be true to ourselves, not only as individuals, nourishing our outside interests, hobbies and pastimes, but also as family members, helping our spouses to bring up our children and supporting each other.

However, what we are often not prepared for, let alone expect, is the spectre of failing health, both physical and emotional, in ourselves and in our families. Women doctors may have to face the possibility of suddenly finding themselves the sole bread-winner when widowed prematurely, or when husbands lose their jobs. Disagreements within the practice are anticipated and expected, but the reality is almost always far more stressful than anticipated. Realising that something has had a greater than anticipated effect on us can, of course, bring its own stresses, and these continued waves, far from losing their impact as they move away from the central stress, retain a surprising force. Yet most of us will somehow survive all of this, deriving some sort of satisfaction from engaging in the struggle, and even showing off our battle scars with pride. But there is a price to be paid and for a significant number of us the struggle will prove too much. None of us can be, or indeed are, prepared for this. Within the struggle, are we prepared, and indeed do we expect, to have to reach out to our colleagues who are struggling? Do I really want somebody else's problems? However, in the nature of partnerships, I am sure that many people recognise their own responsibility to colleagues, and with the increasing openness within practices, there does seem to be an expectation that at some stage in our careers we will find ourselves anxious to reach out to colleagues who are in trouble. Rather than being an expectation of stress, I believe that this should become, increasingly, a source of reassurance.

It has been our experience in our practice that regular appraisals do provide an opportunity to examine these issues and create the appropriate setting for strategic planning. Whether we get it right is another matter!

Age 6: approaching retirement

I have intentionally cast a very broad overview of the third, fourth and fifth ages, allowing them to merge one into the other, as to make too sharp a distinction is, I believe, artificial. Preparation for the sixth age, the early days of retirement, is another matter and GPs approaching this age find their lives brought sharply into focus. Nearing retirement, what sort of shape do we expect to be in and what is the expectation of stress, at what should be a most fulfilling time for us?

How could the interactive model be applied? I do not presume to know if this could work, but there are real issues relating to continuing personal development in retirement, reflecting on the achievement of a career of service in general practice and looking critically at the health of the practice from which the GP is retiring.

Sorting out the practical issues in an orderly and agreeable way is vital and potentially very stressful. Saying goodbye to patients, colleagues and staff, handing over to an incoming partner and setting the finances straight often obscure the emotional impact of retirement. On the one hand, the sense of pride and relief of making it to retirement; on the other, a new lease of life beckoning, with all that free time!

Personal development never stops and retirement provides the opportunity to spend more time on oneself and on one's family. And yet leaving a professional career such as general practice represents a very real loss that none of us can know until we actually experience it. Grieving for that loss can come as a body blow and we are all sadly familiar with the sudden death of recently retired colleagues. Not much is written about this. Is it 'over the top' to speculate that retired GPs may die of a broken heart? For many GPs their careers have been like a long love affair and the reasons that it has to end may be unclear. Some certainly choose to retire in accordance with the practice agreement; some choose to retire early; others may choose to go on working, either as locums, with all the attendant pressures that brings, or within their practices. The change in status is undeniable and I am not sure we really do adequately value the contributions that GPs in this age can make. For some, invitations to be involved in related professional activity, such as professional counselling, teaching, lecturing, etc., can be a sustaining lifeline. Again, rather like the registrar, this can be a very isolating time for an older doctor. Who is on hand to help should the need arise? This is an area that certainly needs researching and my intention here has not been to set out a blueprint, but simply to provoke thought.

Age 7: the final age

The last scene that ends this strange and eventful history has but one exception – to live out our lives to the end as anyone else hopes to, with some happiness and health, hoping to retain our dignity and not to have to endure too much suffering. I have no model on which to base considerations of the stresses of this age and believe that it would be impertinent to try.

Much of what I have written is clearly applicable to many other careers in the caring professions, but much of what we are learning about stress within the career of general practice comes from the experience of looking after patients who have turned to their GPs for help. It is clear that many of our patients acknowledge this and, I believe, are showing their willingness to try to address these stresses within a co-operative and mutually supportive relationship.

Acknowledgements

I am indebted to my partners, Rosemary Lane and Dennis Cox, for their help.

11 Caring for colleagues as patients: how to help others handle stress

John Mitchell

Registration

One way an established GP can help a colleague new to a general practice in his area is to welcome him at an early opportunity and discuss the options for his future healthcare. GP registrars often discuss the advisability or inadvisability of registering with a partner and most now see the conflict of interest that may arise. It may be that if GPs move to a rural location that they may have to register with a GP some way distant. GPs should be open to registering doctors 'out of their practice' areas but be mindful that there may be difficulties for other members of the primary healthcare team, especially visiting community nurses and health visitors.

Early consultation

Whether a GP is taking another doctor onto his list as a new patient, or taking over a list with doctor patients on it, it is advisable to meet early to establish a relationship, build up a position of trust, assess present health and discuss future help-seeking strategies. The initial assessment might include the following.

- Who is registering: the new GP alone or, additionally, the doctor's partner and children?
- Where is he/she living: is this a short-term or long-term address, and in which practice is he/she working?
- How is he/she living? Is he/she involved in the out-of-hours service? Is he/she full- or part-time and what does he/she do to relax and spend leisure time? Drinking and smoking habits should be noted along with any self-medication.
- What aspirations does the GP have for the future and how does the GP see these being fulfilled?
- Practice agreements: has the practice a practice agreement on sickness leave – is the new GP adequately protected for locum insurance and have discussions taken place about practice contingency plans, in the event of long-term sickness?
- Has the GP any immediate health concerns? Is he/she fully immunised, especially against hepatitis B, and in good health? Is there any family history of which the doctor physician should be aware?

A discussion might then take place about future consultations and how they should be arranged. The options are for the doctor patient to use the surgery like any other patient or for him/her to contact the GP directly to negotiate a mutually convenient time.

Robin Steel, in a personal communication, pointed out that looking after doctors and their families is never easy but that there are a number of things that a doctor physician and doctor patient can do to make it easier, including the following.

- Doctor physician
  - see your patient in optimal circumstances
  - establish that you have your patient's trust
  - ask about self-medication
  - ask about self-diagnosis
  - veto any deviations from established procedures
  - try to speak to a relative if your doctor patient agrees, to expand the history and explain.

- Doctor patient
  - trust your GP; you must feel comfortable enough to discuss sensitivities and problems
  - never mention a symptom to a specialist without prior discussion with your GP
  - never take any medicines that a lawyer could not purchase over the counter
  - consult by appointment
  - meticulously follow rituals and protocols set for non-doctor patients.

Consultations for illness in surgery

Whether the consultation is for physical or mental illness, it is likely to be a complex affair. The requisites for a successful conclusion for the doctoring GP are an open approach, time, sensitivity and understanding. GPs are reluctant patients, who tend to consult as a last resort. It is likely that they have made a self-diagnosis and most will have self-medicated with prescriptions after some sort of fashion. The consulting GP may have scanty and incomplete notes and will need to clarify information offered, with which he is not altogether familiar.

Doctor–doctor consultations are also likely to be potentially tense because of two other dynamics: first, the GP may feel undermined by the possible superior knowledge of his colleague patient and, secondly, the GP will want to justify the trust his colleague is investing in him.

The consultation for stress

The agenda for the consultation must cover:

- symptoms or presenting problems, their duration and any precipitating factors

- the doctor patient's own ideas, concerns and expectations
- the effects of the illness on the doctor, his or her family, his or her practice and on individual relationships; remember, doctors are self-employed and many worry about the effects of any illness on future life assurance and sickness insurance policies
- past and family history of stress, depression and other mental illness, including suicide
- lifestyle history – remember, 1 doctor in 15 is alcohol dependent
- physical examination.

The GP may need time to make a diagnosis, which may be stress, anxiety, phobic illness, depression or a combination of these. The diagnosis should be stated, put in perspective and agreed, as this will form the basis of the management plan.

Management plan

The management plan will involve advice on several issues, but before running through the advice, the doctor GP would probably do well to ask himself what he would like doing for him if he were the patient. Advice might include the following.

- The need for **further investigations** – to exclude physical illness (remember to discuss the practicalities of arranging these).
- **Work.** A decision will have to be made with regard to time off work. Many GPs will find this advice hard to take and the doctoring GP may have to adopt a more paternalistic approach to ensure that his advice is followed. Practical issues of how to communicate with the practice and practice agreement details will need to be addressed.
- **Stress management advice.** There are many publications detailing the nature and management of stress – the experienced doctor GP will have his favourite easily to hand, to run

Table 11.1 Advice offered in the Stress Syndrome Foundation leaflet, *How to Prevent Stress in Everyday Life*

1	Plan your day
2	Give yourself satisfaction
3	Be realistic: you are not superhuman
4	Know your concentration span and energy curve
5	Learn to delegate
6	Try to maintain a balanced system
7	It is mature to say no
8	Find something in your work to enjoy
9	Laughing is tension-relaxing
10	Take your foot off the accelerator

through and lend to his patient. For example, the Stress Syndrome Foundation published an excellent leaflet several years ago (Table 11.1).

- **Medication**. Consider antidepressant or short-term anxiolytic medication and give the same advice concerning the pros and cons as you would any other patient.
- **Referrals**. A decision will have to be made as to whether or not to enlist the help of the local mental health team. It may be preferable to organise care away from the local area and perhaps on a private basis. Lists of private counsellors can be readily obtained these days. Personal contact with the provider is desirable, but a detailed referral letter essential.
- **Follow-up**. Fixed arrangements for follow-up must be defined. Many doctor GPs may feel that the best approach is to visit at home, to allow input from those at home.

Caring for doctors perceived to be suffering from stress but not seeking help

Doctors within or without a partnership may, through their own direct observations or through feedback from others, perceive that a colleague is suffering from stress and its consequences, without the colleague accepting that he or she has a problem.

This situation is extremely difficult to address, but it must be addressed, rather than confronted.

In the first instance the 'doctor' GP must choose a good time to sit down with the 'patient' GP and, in a supportive way, ask whether he or she is quite well. This may be enough to 'open' a situation out, but more likely the 'patient' GP might deny problems. It is then necessary for the doctor GP to feed back his observations, seeking explanation and offering to help. It may be that the doctor GP should offer to contact the 'patient' GP's own doctor to arrange an appointment. Alternatively, other outside agencies could be mentioned, including the following.

- **BMA Counselling**, a service for members and their families. Open 24 hours a day to discuss personal, emotional and work-related problems; free except for telephone calls, charged at local rates. Tel.: 0645 200169.
- **National Counselling Service for Sick Doctors**. Open to doctors who are concerned about their own health or that of a colleague, offering confidential advice from senior doctors in all branches of the profession – accessed by phone (Tel.: 020 7935 5982). The caller is not required to give his or her name or any clinical details. The caller will be given the name of an appropriate adviser.

Caring for the unwilling ill doctor

Doctors now have a clear responsibility to report a colleague if they suspect that he or she has a health problem that may put patients at risk. Indeed, failure to act may render them vulnerable to a charge of serious professional misconduct. In such a situation the concerned doctor would do well to first consult the secretary of his local LMC, to see what influence he can bring to bear on the sick

GP. Alternatively, the concerned doctor could consult his defence organisation. Advice and publications are very readily available (for example, from the Medical Protection Societies and MDU).

The first formal step that the concerned doctor may take with regard to a sick unwilling GP is to refer him to the Complaints Officer of his/her employing health authority. The problem will probably then be referred to the health authority Medical Adviser who may act informally or who may suggest formal referral to the health authority Reference Committee. On convening, the Reference Committee has a number of management options, including:

1 no action
2 asking the Medical Adviser to make contact with the GP to discuss further
3 the 'three wise men' approach – clinical governance lead/LMC chairman/GP trainer
4 the Performance Review Committee
5 the Discipline Committee (time-limited and must relate to alleged breach of terms of service)
6 referral to the GMC
7 referral to the police.

A second formal step that the concerned doctor may take is referral to the GMC. Such a measure would inevitably not be taken lightly and not without much soul searching, but should, hopefully, be seen as being constructive in the longer term. The GMC would then decide on an appropriate plan to address the poorly performing doctor.

Medical students and registrars

There is now wide acceptance that the concepts of stress, its causes and its management should be taught and discussed throughout the medical curriculum. Medical students and registrars must build up their own strategies for handling the stress that they encounter during their training, and which they can fall back on in their chosen careers. Strategies that postgraduates have developed, with the backing of their colleagues, include mentoring, Balint-style peer groups and stress management courses.

Useful phone numbers

- BMA 24-hour counselling service: 0645 200169
- National Counselling Service for Sick Doctors: 020 7935 5982
- Overseas Doctors Associations Health Counselling Panel: 0161 236 5594
- Sick Doctors Trust National Helpline for Addicted Physicians: 01252 345 163
- Drinkline/National Alcohol Helpline: London, 020 7332 0202; rest of UK, 0345 320202
- GMC Fitness To Practice Division: 020 7580 7642
- Doctors Support Network: 020 7727 3738
- Royal Medical Benevolent Fund: 020 8540 9194/5
- Centre for Stress Management: 020 8293 4114
                                                                     020 8853 1122
- British Association for Counselling: 01788 550899

12 The stress of complaints

Liz Bingham

There is no doubt that making or receiving a complaint is an extremely stressful experience. Complaints are often the first topic of conversation whenever doctors gather together. How might we be able to harness the nervous energy generated by a complaint and turn it from a wholly negative experience in which the doctor and patient lose, into something more positive for both?

Research has shown that a majority of GPs initially feel out of control, shocked and panicky when one of their patients complains about them. They also feel a sense of indignation towards patients generally, and I guess most of us can identify with those emotions. It is almost like a bereavement. After the first shock, many of us feel angry, depressed; some, even suicidal. There are conflicts around professional identity, clinical competence and towards our family and friends, as well as conflict associated with the management of the complaint. Even after resolution of a complaint we often look back on it as a negative experience which may prompt us to resort to inappropriate defensive practice, and some of us even to leave general practice altogether. What a gloomy picture!

But, all is not lost. A small minority of GPs do find that a complaint has been a learning experience, or they appear to develop some immunity to complaints. Are there lessons we can learn to prevent complaints blighting our lives? What are some of the potential strategies for coping?

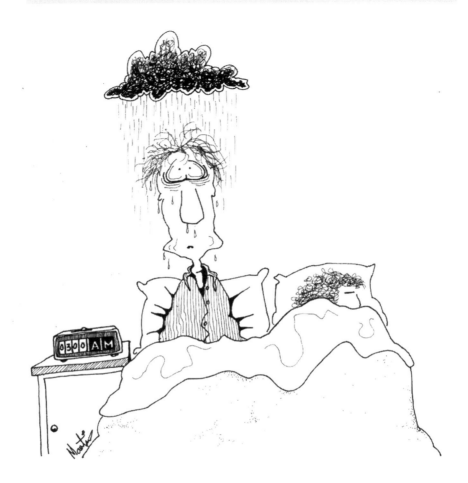

Prevention: listening

There may be ways of consulting with patients which minimise the risk of a complaint being made. The importance of listening to the patients' story cannot be overemphasised. I have had the experience of hearing the stories of a lot of patients who have made complaints about their medical care. Many of them could have been avoided had their doctor heard (properly heard) the story that was being related. One thing that really upsets patients is if they think they have told their doctor some vital piece of information, and think that their doctor has ignored them. Sometimes they have, but more usually their doctor has simply not understood what they were talking about, or they have not understood what the doctor was talking about.

We are all busier than ever before, but even if listening consultations take a little longer, the pay-off is probably worth it. The consequences of ignoring the patients' stories are potentially dire. At best they will need to come back to try to attract our attention to their story; at worst, we may not appreciate what is being related, may fail to interpret the meaning of an important history and, as a result, may make a mistake that harms a patient or leads to a complaint, with all the heartache that either event implies. We could get an awful lot of listening to patients' narratives into the time we may have to spend trying to resolve a complaint. There will, however, always be some complaints. If all the predictions are to be believed, society will become more consumer oriented and the numbers of complaints will rise. What can we do to make the hurt and damage less? Imagine what life might be like if we had less fear of complaints. Let us try to discover whether it is possible to prevent ourselves from regarding a complaint as a fundamental challenge to our professional identity. If we really can learn to transform our attitude to complaints, think of the rewards.

Getting over the shock and panic: TEARS

- **Talking.** It is vitally important that if ever a GP receives a complaint he or she avoids becoming isolated. Talk to someone. Preferably both family and colleagues, so that they can all understand that you are worried. While you are telling them, be frank about how worried you are. Obviously this will vary, but they need to know so they can give any necessary support, rather than thinking your bad temper, moods or depression are caused by something they did!

- **Evaluating.** Once that important step has been taken, try to evaluate, calmly, exactly what the complaint is about. Try to understand where the patient is coming from, and be brutally honest with yourself. Is this a mistake you have made, or is there a simple explanation?
- **Accepting.** If you have made a mistake, this does not mean that you are a bad doctor, but it does mean that there may be something you need to apologise for. Apologies are hard to make. There is the fear that an apology means admitting negligence, or that there is an associated loss of face, but time and again, patients who have been unlucky enough to be the victim of a medical mistake say that they genuinely appreciated a full and honest apology. A quick, spontaneous apology can sometimes stop any further action.
- **Raging.** It can help to let off steam to some one you really trust. Just make sure that it is not the complainant, and make sure that you do not take any action or write any letters until you have had time to calm down. A lot of anger is generated by a belief that many complainants are simply malicious or vindictive, and indeed this is so in a few cases. Even then, overt anger will seldom help. Whether you feel angry, afraid or depressed, the effect these emotions have serves to hinder the constructive resolution of the complaint by almost paralysing the doctor's communication skills. Patients are left with defensive and incomplete responses, which do nothing to help them understand the answers to questions they are posing. Or they get no response at all.
- **Sharing.** If you try to manage a complaint alone, it can feel extremely lonely, which only adds to the distress. It does not have to be like that. Every practice should have a complaints team and it is important to let colleagues help from the beginning. A practice manager can take a step back from the clinical issues, and take a more independent view as well as contributing a lay perspective. The practice may have a patient participation group who could help, and there should be

another partner who could handle clinical aspects of a complaint. It is helpful and important to try to answer complaints as impartially as possible. If the practice finds it difficult to achieve that (either because there are several partners involved in the complaint, or because you are single handed), consider asking a neighbouring practice, or a conciliator, to help out. Above all, contact your defence organisation for support and advice, and then take it!

Getting back in control: TRADE

One of the bad things about receiving a complaint is the feeling of being out of control. Let's look at ways of seizing the initiative and getting back in control.

- **Timetable.** Any formal complaint to the practice, whether written or oral, has to be handled within the NHS complaints procedures and, hopefully, fully resolved through local resolution. A timetable is laid down, which you must adhere to. The complaint must be acknowledged in writing within three working days, and a full response should be given within 10 working days. If you set out to achieve the deadlines laid down in the guidlines, rather than delay in the hope that the complainant will get fed up and go away, you keep in control, and can avoid additional hassle. If there are special reasons why a complete response cannot be given, such as key personnel being on holiday, or medical records not available, say so straight away, but again set a new, and realistic, timetable and stick to it.
- **Responses.** When you have completed your investigation to establish all the facts, write a really full reply. It is vital to cover each separate point that the complainant makes. Some might seem trivial to you, but if a patient has gone to the trouble of writing a grievance down, or approaching their doctor or practice personally to complain, you can be certain that they

think it important. One thing guaranteed to make a complaint run and run is to give the impression that you are trying to avoid answering part of it. This is so often interpreted as feeling or being 'guilty'. When you have finished writing, send a draft to your defence organisation, preferably by fax so that you do not build in any unnecessary delays.

- **Actions**. Most complainants do not want blood, or even compensation, but an assurance that if anything has gone wrong, action will be taken to prevent recurrences. Sometimes, even when nothing has gone wrong, an investigation of a complaint will reveal problems in your administration or systems. If there is anything you can tell the patient about any improvements you intend to make as a result of their comments, try to tell them. It gives them a warm glow, and helps you to keep in control by making sure that any changes you need to make are driven by you, and not forced on you by outside agencies.

- **Defence**. One worry that many GPs have is that complaints make them practise 'defensively' by ordering unnecessary investigations or X-rays, or making inappropriate referrals. This further undermines their belief in their own professionalism. I don't believe that this form of defence is at all helpful. If a test, X-ray or referral is inappropriate, it will be no protection at all. What is a superb defence is the ability to justify your own decisions, and to be able to show that you really did do enough to back up your clinical judgement. If you have good contemporary records, and a logical plan of action based on well-recognised current practice to support your account of events, a complaint against you is unlikely to go far. Even if a complaint is pursued through several stages, you can almost relax.
  - GOOD RECORDS
    - (i) History (quote any significant words, for example 'headache – the worst I've ever had'). It is particularly important to cover the full range of questions you ask when recording a telephone consultation.

(ii) Objective assessment, including any examination or investigation (briefly note actions taken and, for each, whether there were positive or negative findings).

(iii) Assessment (your working diagnosis and differential diagnoses if you have several ideas). A note of what you shared with the patient.

(iv) Plan (treatment prescribed, plans for follow-up, referral, etc., and what plans you made with the patient in case anything unexpected happened).

- **Explanation.** Where you need to give an explanation, it is important to avoid medical abbreviations, technical words and jargon. Wherever possible, refer to your notes made at the time, but explain what they mean. It is pointless to say to a worried complainant 'I can assure you that I examined your mother's chest and heart carefully; look, it says here CVS/RS NAD'. If your notes recorded more detail about what you did to reach the conclusion that there was nothing wrong in the cardiovascular or respiratory system, it would help your explanation enormously.

Recovery: VALUE

- **Valuing skills.** The challenge of learning how to consult better, to listen, to explain, and to check on your patient's understanding is difficult, but rewarding and valued. How much better if GPs learn how to handle complaints so that they can come to their practice confident in the knowledge that they have learnt to cope emotionally, and to communicate with dissatisfied patients coolly and effectively, rather than being constantly in dread of receiving a complaint.
- **Analysis.** It may help to take a step back and analyse how communications have failed, and try to make a plan to address any misunderstandings, especially during conciliation.

- **Learning.** The skills needed to resolve complaints can be taught. The expertise is there. Countless commercial companies have customer service departments. The best have highly skilled customer service managers who train their staff to understand that complaints are not directed personally at them, to respond courteously until the customer is calm and then to resolve the problem. We have learnt other management skills from industry before. Why not these? They are all about connection with the patient, but the emotional impact of the complaint on a doctor is a powerful inhibitor of effective communication. It has become a recognised part of the curriculum to teach consultation skills; why not complaints handling? There is a real and justifiable pride in becoming a skilled communicator. Next time you have to return something faulty, or send back a meal in a restaurant, watch and listen carefully. How is your complaint handled? How does that make you feel? Did you learn anything that might help you to respond to someone who complains to you?

- **Understanding.** Another approach that might have something to contribute is cognitive therapy. There is good evidence that it is effective in the management of depression. If the reaction of doctors to a complaint does so often resemble a depressive illness, it would make sense to explore whether a similar psychological approach might be of value. One cognitive approach could be to challenge whether the emotional response – that a complaint cuts at the heart of a doctor's professional image – stands up in reality. Ask a few questions. Do you despise other colleagues who have had a complaint made against them? How many patients have expressed gratitude, approval, support? How many more of them are there than those who have ever complained? What evidence do you have that, on the whole, you have kept up to date and are proud of the job you do? Be honest, has the complaint told you something important that really does need fixing? In reality, there will be a great mass of positive feedback that you can identify.

You can use this sort of analysis to put a complaint into perspective. Of course, you need to answer it and try to put things right; but each event, good or bad, must be allowed equal weight. For the vast majority of GPs the positive feedback will outweigh the negative by a big margin.

- **Equanimity.** The aim of this exercise is to try to regain peace of mind, to value your own work and allow you to incorporate the professional handling of complaints into a thoroughly professional framework for practice. Once complaint handling becomes a valued part of the culture, a complaint stops being a threat, but becomes another opportunity to demonstrate expertise.

13 Conclusion

David Haslam

Is it all worth it? Having read through an entire book dealing with the stresses of being a GP, is it really worth going on? Wouldn't it be easier to give it all up and find something else to do – such as defusing unexploded bombs or professional boxing?

A tiny minority of GPs will realise that they have made an error in their choice of career, but for most of us general practice has the potential to be one of the most rewarding, fascinating and worthwhile jobs. GPs are greatly appreciated by most patients, are reasonably well paid and can end each day feeling that time spent was generally worthwhile. We are faced with a never-ending variety of different problems – no one knows what the next minute may bring. Once we have taken control of the job, and learnt how to control our stress, then general practice can be tremendously enjoyable.

It really is worth persevering. As Kevork Hopayian wrote in his chapter, the reason that many GPs moan that general practice is boring and full of trivia is because they have set their sights too low. They confine themselves to the most facile work and miss the many challenges that our job can bring.

Also remember that research has shown that the GPs who become most stressed are likely to be more caring and patient-centred than many of their colleagues. General practice is easy to do badly. Indeed, far from being the soft option of medical practice, it is probably the hardest speciality to do really well. GPs have a great deal to be proud of.

A final tip. One of the rules of general practice is that the people for whom we do the most are those least likely to thank us, and those for whom we do the least are the most grateful. Nowadays, British general practice is generally so good that our patients often take us for granted. So when you do get the rare thank-you letters or notes, don't throw them away. Keep them in a file, and when the job threatens to become too stressful, have a look through your file. People do appreciate us. What we do is worthwhile. While you look at the letters, ask yourself how many thank-you letters our politicians and health service administrators receive. Which job would you rather be doing?

If you are feeling stressed, you will now realise that you are certainly not alone. If times have been hard, then I do hope that this book has helped you to find ways of coping, surviving and enjoying your life and your work again. You spend your life caring for your patients. Now is the time to start caring for yourself.

Appendix: Contacts, useful references and further reading

IK Campbell

Contacts

Below is a list of organisations, services, associations and individuals willing to help general practitioners with problems with stress.

British Doctors and Dentists Group
Tel.: 020 7487 4445
Rescues and rehabilitates alcoholic and addicted doctors, dentists and their families. Supports the sick doctor or dentist, giving confidential help and advice through a local recovering doctor or dentist.

Cheviot Consultancy Ltd
Heron House, 5 Heron Square, Richmond, Surrey TW9 1EL, UK
Tel.: 020 8332 1842/Fax: 020 8332 2482
Professional stress management. The services available include stress audits, stress management training, coaching, consultancy, counselling skills training and 'train the trainer' courses.

CONTACT
Tel.: 0121 5580278
Free, independent clinical psychology and counselling service to all NHS doctors and dentists in the West Midlands region. This is aimed at helping doctors and dentists to live and work more confidently and effectively.

COPE

Contact: Dr Malcolm Price, Scheme Co-ordinator Tel.: 0117 935 4447 or Dr Elizabeth Robinson, Avon Health Authority's primary care medical adviser.

COPE is a confidential counselling scheme for GPs in Avon. The health authority set up a support system for GPs in 1996 with the backing of the LMC and funding from the health authority. It gives GPs directed access to GP helpers, psychologists, counsellors and psychiatrists.

Counselling in Primary Care Trust

Suite 3a, Majestic House, High Street, Staines, Middlesex TW18 4DG, UK
Tel.: 01784 441782

GP Care

Dovedale Counselling Ltd, 2 Dovedale Studios, 465 Battersea Park Road, London SW11 4LN, UK
Tel.: 020 7228 6768

Schemes in Bedfordshire, Buckinghamshire, Hertfordshire, Lambeth, Southwark, Lewisham and other local schemes in Lothian and Bolton. These are confidential self-referral counselling services delivered locally by qualified, professional counsellors. Unlimited telephone support is provided, backed by limited-session face-to-face counselling.

GP Stress Factory

Contact: Dr Chris Manning, General Practitioner, Teddington, Middlesex

Set up by Dr Chris Manning in 1994, it aims to help grassroots GPs reduce stress in a fun atmosphere.

MIND
Granta House, 15–19 Broadway, London E15 4BQ, UK
Tel.: 020 8519 2122
Apart from its general activities as a charity for the promotion of mental health, MIND produces a range of relevant information leaflets, publications and factsheets. Particularly helpful is a factsheet entitled *Stress at Work*. This contains topics on the causes of stress and what can help relieve stress.

National Association for Staff Support (NASS) in healthcare
9 Caradon Close, Woking, Surrey GU21 3DU, UK

Staffordshire GP Support Scheme
Contact: Professor Ruth Chambers, Primary Care Development, School of Health, Staffordshire University, Leek Road, Stoke-on-Trent ST4 2DF, UK
Offers GPs one-to-one counselling with a psychologist, as well as stress management and assertiveness skills workshops.

Stress Management Training Institute (incorporating Relaxation for Living)
Foxhills, 30 Victoria Avenue, Shanklin, Isle of Wight PO37 6LS, UK
Tel.: 01983 868166
A charity devoted to promoting effective forms of stress management and relaxation. Produces self-help resources (including leaflets, audio cassettes and videotapes), home-based support, professional courses and additional services.

The British Confederation of Psychotherapists
37 Mapesbury Road, London NW2 4HJ, UK
Tel.: 020 8830 5173
For a directory of details of registered psychotherapists.

The British Holistic Medical Association
59 Lansdowne Place, Hove, East Sussex BN3 1FL, UK
Tel.: 01273 725951
Information about holistic approaches to treatment and healing.

The Group-Analytic Practice
88 Montagu Mansions, London W1H 1LF, UK
Tel.: 020 7935 3103/020 7935 3085
This private organisation provides comprehensive psychotherapeutic assessment and has the ability to refer on to a wide range of psychotherapies and psychotherapists according to need. The practice offers group analysis, short- and long-term individual psychotherapy or psychoanalysis, work with psychosomatic disorders, long-term contact and support, if needed, and will respond rapidly in urgent cases.

The Institute for Complementary Medicine
PO Box 194, London SE16 1QZ, UK
Provides details of a range of therapies, which may be useful in stress management. Also has a list of organisations, which may offer a variety of approaches. Send a stamped addressed envelope for details.

The National Counselling Service for Sick Doctors
Tel.: 020 7306 3272/020 7935 5982 (9.30 a.m.–4.30 p.m. Mon–Fri)
Confidential independent advisory service for sick doctors, which is supported by the medical Royal Colleges, the Joint Consultants Committee, the BMA and other professional bodies. Set up in 1985, it offers general advice and information. A network of advisers return calls from sick doctors or those worried about a sick doctor and refer sick doctors to counsellors as appropriate.

The Promis Recovery Centre and the Promis Counselling Centre
2A Cromwell Place, London SW7 2JE, UK
Tel.: 020 7581 8222
A professional, confidential counselling service for those who have problems with alcohol, food, gambling, nicotine, drugs or other compulsive behaviours. Also has a 24-hour crisis line.

The Stress Counselling Service for Doctors
Tel.: 0645 200169
Run by Care Assist, this scheme was launched in April 1996 for all doctors. This is a counselling service that is available 24 hours a day. Callers are able to speak to trained non-medical counsellors. The service offers direct ongoing support or referral to specialised services.

Useful references

Appleton K, House A and Dowell A (1998) A survey of job satisfaction, sources of stress and psychological symptoms among general practitioners in Leeds. *Br J Gen Pract.* **48**(428): 1059–63.

Bailey S (1982) The management of personal stress. *J Assoc Course Organisers.* **3**(2): 93–6.

Branthwaite A and Ross A (1988) Satisfaction and job stress in general practice. *Fam Pract.* **5**(2): 83–93.

Bynoe G (1994) Stress in women doctors. *Br J Hosp Med.* **51**(6): 267–8.

Caplan RP (1994) Stress, anxiety and depression in hospital consultants, general practitioners, and senior health managers. *BMJ.* **309**: 1261–3.

Abstract

A study to measure stress, anxiety and depression in a group of senior health service staff, which concludes that the levels of stress, anxiety and depression in senior doctors and managers in the NHS seem to be high and perhaps higher than expected.

Chambers R (1993) Avoiding burnout in general practice (editorial). *Br J Gen Pract.* **43**(376): 442–3.

Chambers R and Belcher J (1992) Self-reported health care over the past 10 years: a survey of general practitioners. *Br J Gen Pract* **42**: 153–6.

Chambers R and Campbell I (1996) Anxiety and depression in general practitioners: associations with type of practice, fundholding, gender and other personal characteristics. *Fam Pract.* **13**(2): 170–3.

Chambers R and Maxwell R (1996) Helping sick doctors (editorial). *BMJ.* **312**: 722–3.

Chambers R, George V, McNeill A *et al.* (1998) Health at work in the general practice. *Br J Gen Pract.* **48**: 1501–4.

Cooper CL, Rout U and Faragher B (1989) Mental health, job satisfaction and job stress among general practitioners. *BMJ.* **298**: 366–70.

Cox T (1993) *Stress research and stress management: putting theory to work.* HSE Contract Research Report No. 61/1993. HSE, Suffolk.

Cullen J and Sandberg CG (1987) Wellness and stress management programmes – a critical evaluation. *Ergonomics.* **30**: 287–94.

Firth-Cozens J (1997) Predicting stress in general practitioners: 10 year follow-up postal survey. *BMJ.* **315**: 34–5.

Hawkins J (1992) Benefits of stress management groups. *Practitioner.* **236**(1510): 20–3.

Abstract

Stress management techniques can be of great benefit in a variety of physical and psychological conditions. Both relaxation skills and physical exercise can be used to reduce stress levels.

Howie JG, Hopton JL, Heaney DJ *et al.* (1992) Attitudes to medical care, the organisation of work and stress among general practitioners. *Br J Gen Pract.* **42**(358): 181–5.

Abstract

Doctors with a higher patient-centred orientation find their work more stressful. Longer booking intervals remove much of that stress, particularly when doctors' preferred style of consulting requires them to spend more time at individual consultations.

Howie J, Porter M and Heaney D (1993) *General Practitioners: work and stress.* Occasional Paper No. 16. Royal College of General Practitioners, London, pp. 18–29.

Kirwan M and Armstrong D (1995) Investigation of burnout in a sample of British general practitioners. *Br J Gen Pract.* **45**(394): 259–60.

Abstract

This study highlights the need to look at the extent of burnout in young doctors during their training and at those characteristics of part-time general practitioners which might prevent burnout.

Myerson S (1991) Doctors' methods of dealing with 'on going' stress in general practice. *Med Sci Res.* **19**: 267–9.

Ostell A (1991) Coping, problem solving and stress: a framework for intervention strategies. *Br J Med Psychol.* **64**: 11–24.

Post DM (1997) Values, stress and coping among practising family physicians. *Arch Fam Med.* **6**(3): 252–5.

Abstract

Results suggest that assessment of the developmental processes in physician stress and coping is important.

Pullen D, Lonie CE, Lyle DM *et al.* (1995) Medical care of doctors. *Med J Aust.* **162**(9): 481, 484.

Rout U and Rout JK (1994) Job satisfaction, mental health and job stress among general practitioners before and after the new contract – a comparative study. *Fam Pract.* **11**(3): 300–6.

Shatner P (1998) Stress in General Practice. How can GPs cope? *Aust Fam Phys.* **27**(11): 993–8.

Abstract

This paper examines the range of coping strategies available to GPs and suggests several support mechanisms.

Simms J (1997) The evaluation of stress management strategies in general practice: an evidence-led approach. *Br J Gen Pract.* **47**(422): 577–82.

Abstract

Interventions to reduce stress in general practice have been introduced at both an individual and an organisational level, but there is little published evidence of their effectiveness. This paper systematically reviews the literature and reports that the research evidence from stress-management programmes employed with other workforces is equivocal. Results so far suggest that relaxation and cognitive behavioural skills are helpful and that group methods are both more cost-effective and more beneficial than individual counselling.

Spurgeon P, Barwell F and Maxwell R (1995) Types of work stress and implications for the role of general practitioners. *Hlth Serv Manag Res.* **8**(3): 186–97.

Sutherland VJ and Cooper CL (1992) Job stress, satisfaction and mental health among general practitioners before and after introduction of new contract. *BMJ*. **304**: 1545–8.

Sutherland VJ and Cooper C (1993) Identifying distress among general practitioners: predictors, psychological ill-health and job dissatisfaction. *Soc Sci Med.* **37**(5): 575–81.

Wilson A, McDonald P, Hayes L *et al.* (1991) Longer booking intervals in general practice: effects on doctors' stress and arousal. *Br J Gen Pract.* **41**(346): 184–7.

Abstract

It is concluded that longer booking intervals are of psychological advantage to general practitioners.

Further reading

Briggs Myers I and Myers P (1995) *Gifts Differing. Understanding Personality Types.* Davies-Black Publishing, California.

Burnard P (1991) *Coping with Stress in the Health Professions.* Chapman & Hall, London.

Butler G and Hope T (1995) *Manage your Mind. The Mental Health Fitness Guide.* Oxford University Press, Oxford.

Chambers R and Davies M (1999) *What Stress in Primary Care! The Once in a Lifetime Programme that will Help you Control Stress in Your Practice.* RCGP, London.

Chambers R and Maxwell R (1997) *Database of Activities and Initiatives in the UK Associated with Reducing GPs' Stress or Improving the GP's Well-being.* RCGP GP Stress Fellowship, London.

Abstract

One of the tasks of the GP Stress Fellowship Fellows has been to promote good models and initiatives to help reduce GPs' stress and improve their well-being. A database form was distributed to over 300 individuals, and 70 or so were completed. The result is that there are many more support organisations in 1997 than there were in 1995 and the contact details are given in the database.

Chambers R, Coventry K and Clare A (1996) *Survival Skills for GPs: an education pack written and designed especially for general practitioners, in two parts of two 12 hour modules.* Stoke Health Centre, Stoke-on-Trent. (Loose-leaf binder containing four items including one video and two tapes.)

Chambers R (1999) *Survival Skills for GPs.* Radcliffe Medical Press, Oxford.

Charlesworth EA and Nathan RG (1997) *Stress Management – A Comprehensive Guide to Wellness.* Souvenir Press, London.

Abstract

A comprehensive self-help manual that offers a huge range of practical steps that can help to reduce stress. It helps to identify the cause of stress and so learn to channel the tension into a positive source of energy.

Chorlton P (1995) *Staying Fit at Work.* Health Education Authority, London.

Cooper C and Cartwright S (1996) *Mental Health and Stress in the Workplace. A Guide for Employers.* HMSO, London.

Cozens J (1991) *OK 2 Talk Feelings.* BBC Books, London.

Grainger C (1994) *Stress Survival Guide.* BMJ Publishing Group, London.

Hare B (1996) *Be Assertive.* Vermilion, London.

Jones H (1997) *I'm Too Busy to be Stressed.* Hodder and Stoughton, London.

Kirsta A (1986) *The Book of Stress Survival.* Allen & Unwin, London.

Lewis D (1995) *10 Minute Time and Stress Management.* Piatkus, London.

Looker T and Gregson O (1989) *Stresswise. A Practical Guide for Dealing with Stress.* Hodder and Stoughton, London.

McCormick EW (1997) *Surviving Breakdown – A Positive Approach to Coping, Healing and Rebuilding Your Life.* Vermilion, London.

A comprehensive and positive guide, written by a psychotherapist with extensive experience of people in crisis, examining all the relevant topics related to nervous breakdown.

Open University (1992) *Handling Stress.* The Open University, Milton Keynes.

Patel C (1989) *The Complete Guide to Stress Management.* Optima, London.

Walmsley C (1992) *Assertiveness – the Right to be You.* BBC Books, London.

Woodham A (1995) *Beating Stress at Work.* Health Education Authority, London.

Audio Cassettes

Coping with Stress at Work

Feeling Good – How to Feel Better about Yourself (self esteem, assertiveness)

The Relaxation Kit

All available from Wendy Lloyd Audio Productions Ltd, PO Box 1, Wirral, L47 7DD, UK.

Index